Goldenthal Eye Drawing

Diagnostic Imaging

DR. AHUVA GOLDENTHAL

Copyright © 2008 by Dr. Ahuva Goldenthal. 47329-GOLD
Library of Congress Control Number: 2008902802
ISBN: Softcover 978-1-4363-3216-3
Hardcover 978-1-4363-3217-0

All rights reserved. No part of this book may be reproduced or transmitted in any form or by any means, electronic or mechanical, including photocopying, recording, or by any information storage and retrieval system, without permission in writing from the copyright owner.

This book was printed in the United States of America.

To order additional copies of this book, contact:
Xlibris Corporation
1-888-795-4274
www.Xlibris.com
Orders@Xlibris.com

TABLE OF CONTENTS

OBJECTIVES FOR EARLY CHILDHOOD

1. To detect early signs of Kookshrek Anxiety.
2. To detect early academic concerns.
3. To promote and expand artistic skills.
4. Child development.
5. To identify objects.
6. To develop good motor skills.
7. Psycho and academic analysis.
8. To increase sensory awareness.
9. To reverse frightening images to profound realism.

EYE INTELLIGENCE PROFILING FOR EARLY CHILDHOOD

(EIP GOALS)
L____6____L
L____5____L
L___4___L
L__3__L
L__2__L
L_1_L

TODAY'S DATE___/___/_________
NAME: ________________________
D. O B.: ______/______/__________
SEX: (M) (F)
TEL: ( )____________________
ADDRESS: ____________________
____
SCHOOL:______________________

COMMENTS: ______________
____
____
____
____
____
____
____
____
____
____
____

ADVANCED LEVEL

1___2___3___4___5__6__
1ST GRADE ________________6
PRE-1-A ___________________5 A
KG __________________________4
NURSERY __________________3 G
PRE-SCHOOL ______________2
TODDLER__________________1 E
INFANT ____________________0
0__1__2__3__4__5__6__
LEVEL OF ACHIEVEMENT

GEDDI APTITUDE TEST FOR EARLY CHILDHOOD

TODAY'S DATE_____/___/_____

NAME: ____________________ AGE:__________ D. O B.: _______/_____/________

ADDRESS: ____

TEL: (   )_________________ Cell phone   (   )_____/_____/_________

FAX: (   )_________________ Emergency phone (   )_____/_____/_________

GRADE: _____________   SEX: (M) (F)

CURRENT SCHOOL: ____

CONCERNS: ____

PRIMARY PHYSICIAN: ____

ADDRESS: ____

TELEPHONE: (   )_____/_____/______

SCHOOL TEACHER________________________

SCHOOL COUNSELOR______________________

PSYCHOLOGIST _________________________

REFERRED BY___________________________

TELEPHONE: (   )_____/_____/__________

TODAY'S DATE____/____/___

ACADEMIC

1________	16_______	30________	44________	58________	72________
2________	17_______	31________	45________	59________	73________
3________	18_______	32________	46________	60________	74________
4________	19_______	33________	47________	61________	75________
5________	20______	34_______	48________	62________	76________
6________	21_______	35________	49________	63________	77________
7________	a_______	b_______	c_______	d_______	e_______ f_______ g_______
8________	22_______	36________	50________	64________	78________
9________	23_______	37________	51________	65________	79________
10________	24_______	38________	52________	66________	80________
11________	25_______	39________	53________	67________	81________
12________	26_______	40________	54________	68________	82________
13________	27_______	41________	55________	69________	83________
14________	28_______	42________	56________	70________	84________
15________	29_______	43________	57________	71________	85________

TOTAL SCORE_____/_____=______%

ACADEMIC

1

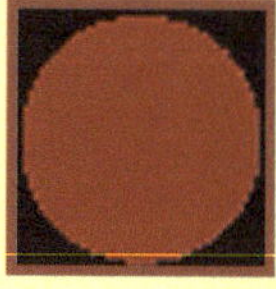

2

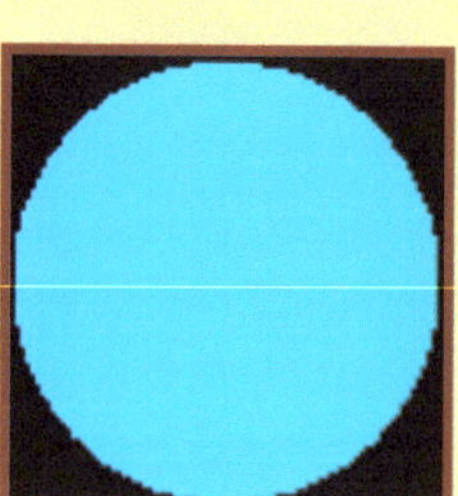

3

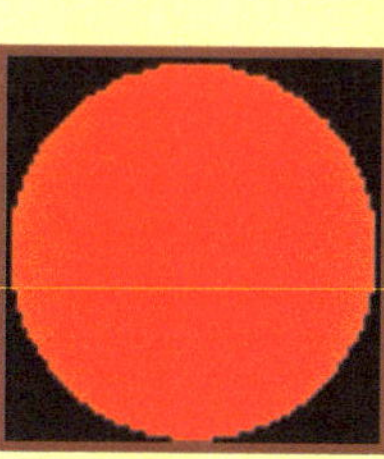

1. Show me the smallest ball? _______________
2. Which ball is blue? _______________________
3. Which ball is your favorite color? _________

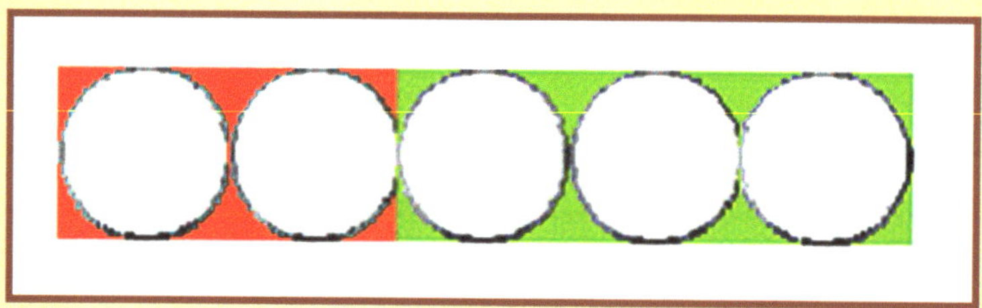

4. How many balls do you see on the red surface? ________
5. How many balls do you see on the green surface? ________
6. How many balls are there all together? ___________________
7. If I take away three balls, how many balls do you have left? ______________________

1 2 3

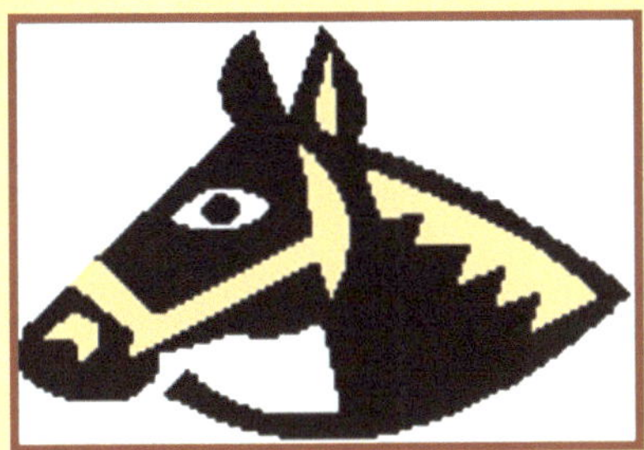
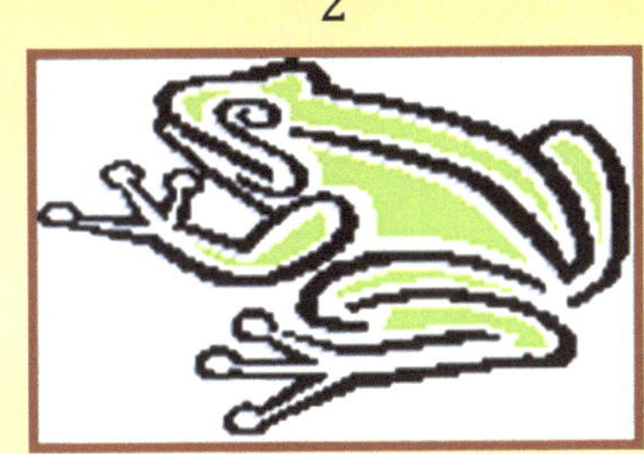
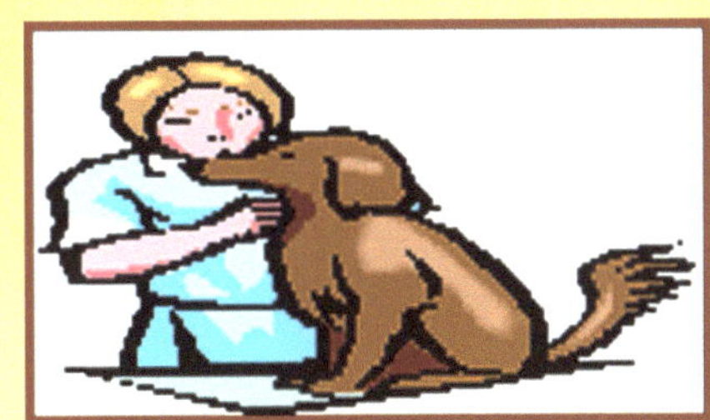

a. Show me the frog. 1 2 3

b. Name the first picture above. ____________

c. Where is the dog? ____________

e. How many animals are there in these pictures? _____

f. And how many people? _____

g. Is the person a boy or a girl? ______________

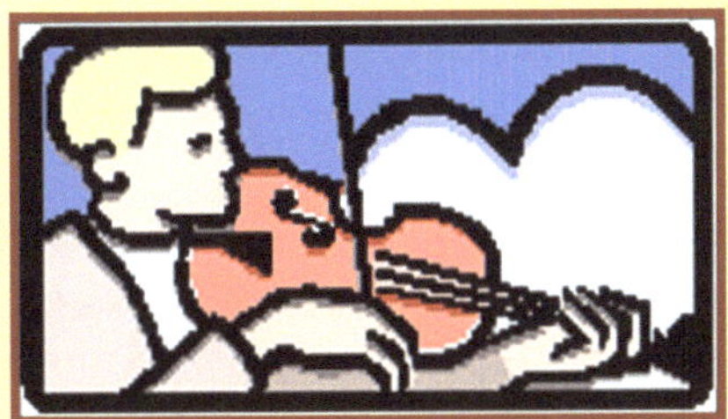

8. What is the man doing? __________________________

9. Do you know what instrument he is playing? ________

10. Can you play? (Y) (N)

11. Would you like to play an instrument? (Y) (N)

12. What is your favorite musical instrument? __________________

13. What is your favorite song? ________________________________

---

1 2 3

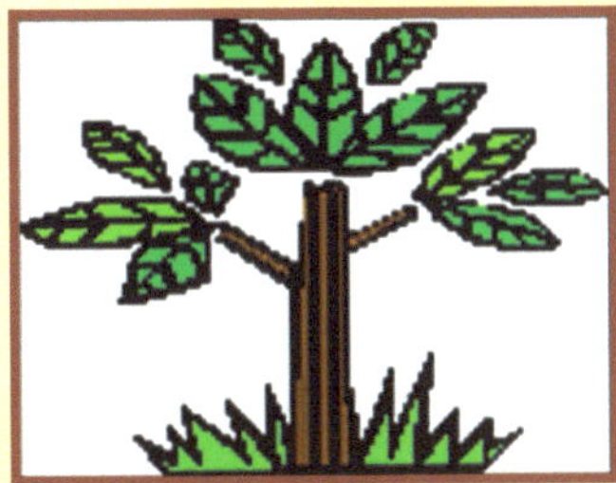
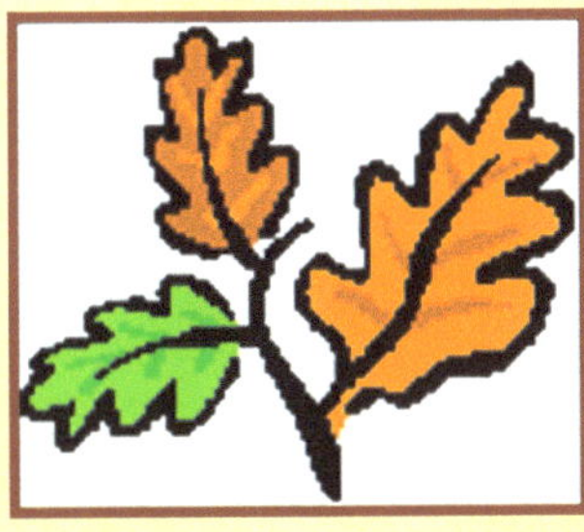
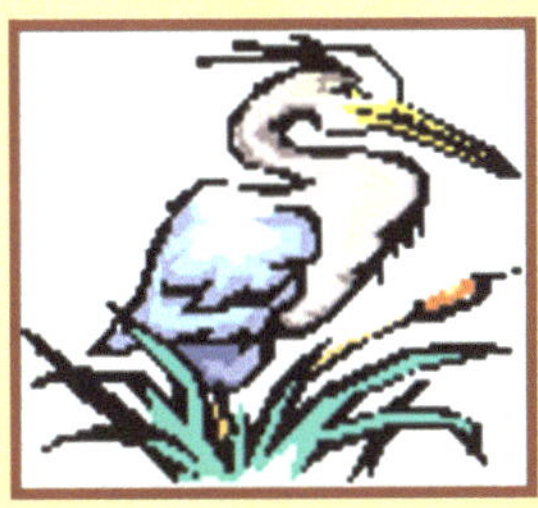

14. Where is the bird? 1 2 3

15. On what is the bird sitting? ____________________________________

16. Show me the tree.____

17. How many leaves grow on the tree? _____________________________

18. Name the picture below. ______________________________

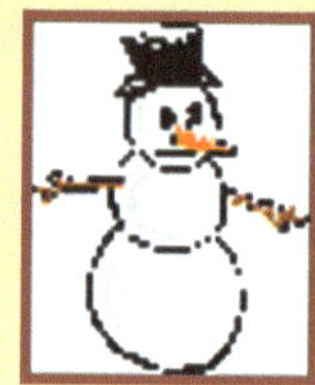

19. How many snowmen are there in number one line? ______________

1 2 3 4

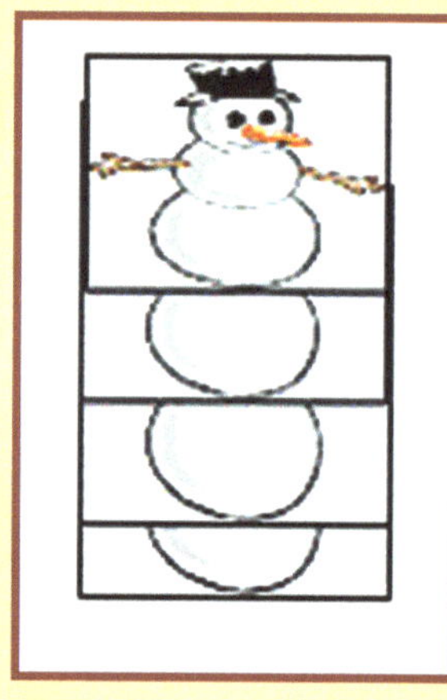

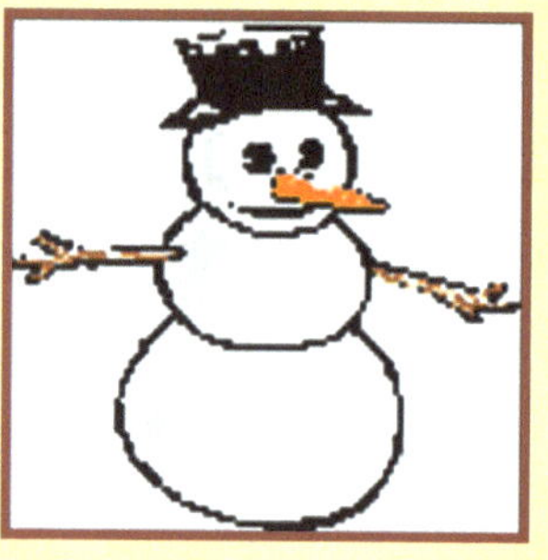

20. Which is the biggest snowman? ______________________
21. Which is the next biggest snowman? ______________________
22. Which is the smallest snowman? ______________________
23. Can you make a snowman? ______________________

SENSORY AWARENESS AND MOTOR SKILLS DEVELOPMENT

24. Let's make a snowman.

Here are the things you can use to make a snowman.

a. A bib so you won't get dirty
b. A plastic to cover the table or a highchair
c. Three sizes of cotton balls
d. Paint, and a small bowl to pour the paint into
e. Orange and black paper
f. Eyes
g. Toothpicks
e. Glue

E y E
On
NUMBERS, LETTERS, AND SHAPES

Left Right

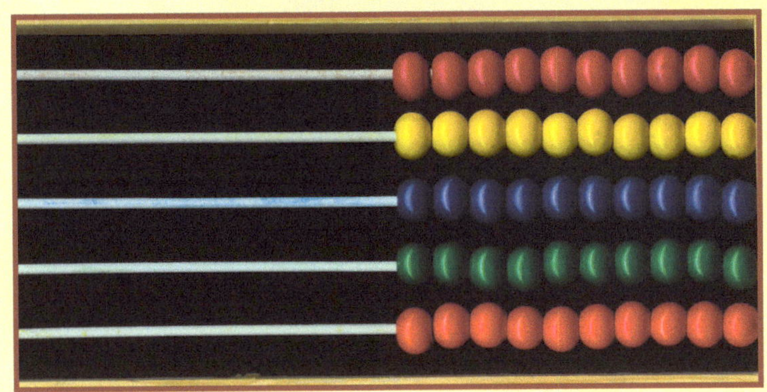

25. Move all the green beads to the left? ________________
26. Keep 4 blue beads to the right, and the rest move to the left. ________________
27. Keep 5 green beads to the left, and the rest move to the right. ________________
28. Move 2 yellow beads to the left, and the rest keep to the right. ________________
29. And now move 2 red to the left, and the rest keep to the right. ________________
30. How many beads are there on the right side? ________________
31. How many beads are there on the left side? ________________
32. Now count them all, and tell me how many beads are there all together. ________________
33. Which of the following blocks does not have a letter?

1 2 3 4 5

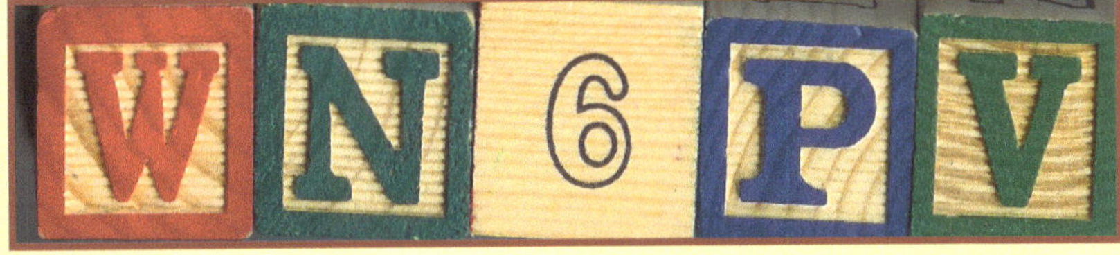

34. Which block is different and how? ________________

1 2 3 4

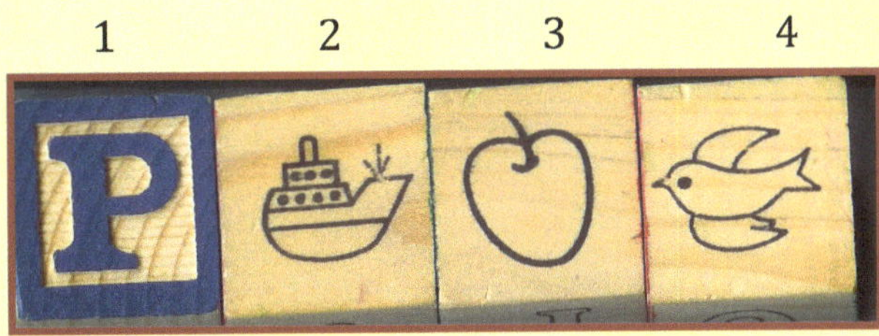

35. Name each picture.

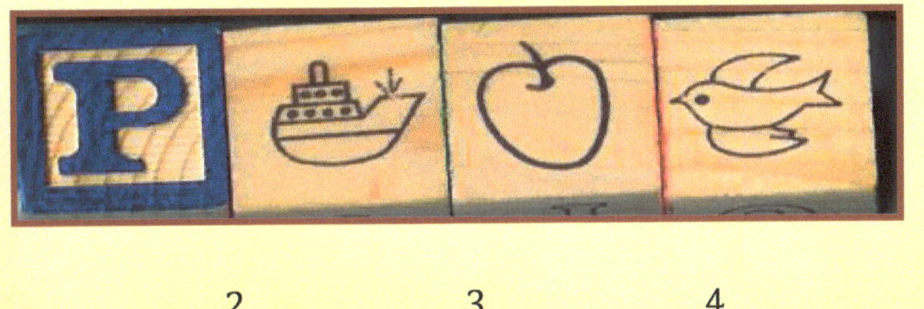

1__________ 2__________ 3__________ 4__________

36. Arrange the letters in order. 1______2______3______4_____5_____

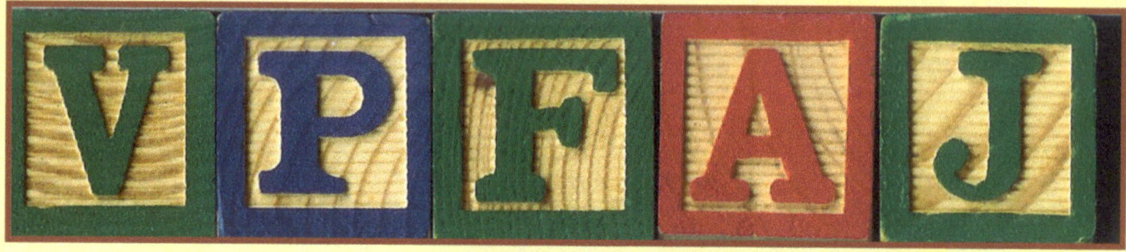

37. Pick the letter W N S G I

___ ___ ___ ___ ___

38. Use these letters to spell the word "wings." ___ ___ ___ ___ ___

39. Pick the letter 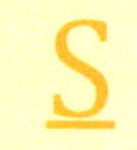 S W I N G

___ ___ ___ ___ ___

40. Now read the word ____________________________.

41. What number is this? 6 5 1 3 __ __ __ __

42. What letter is this? B A F G D S __ __ __ __ __ __ __

43. Correct the mistakes. J K M L N O P Q R S D U V W M Y Z

_ _ _ _ _ _ _ _ _ _ _ _ _ _ _ _ _ _ _ _

44. Name each shape below.

1 2 3 4 5

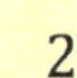

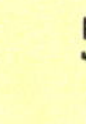

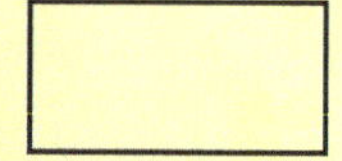

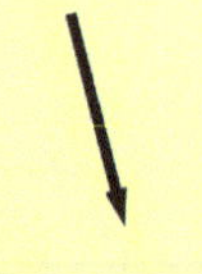

______ ______ ______ ______ ______

45. Which two items have nothing in common?

1 2 3 4 5 6

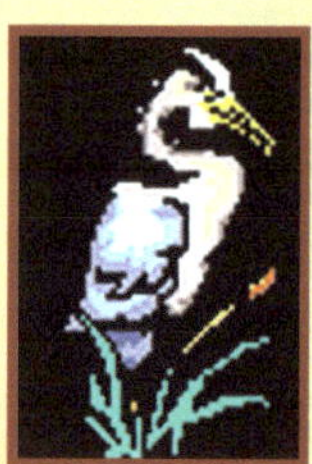

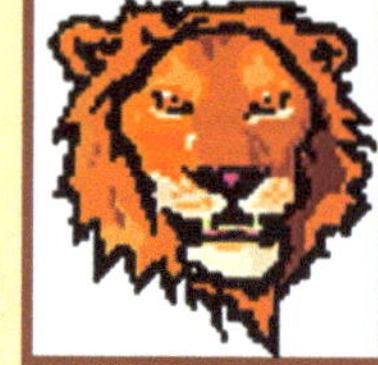

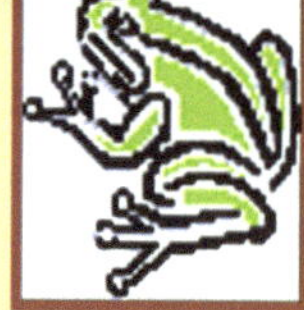

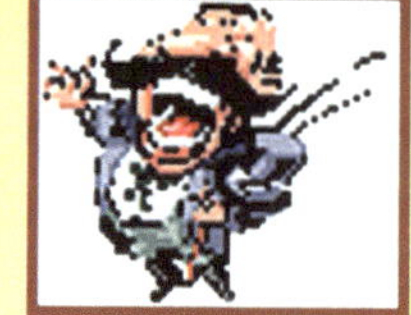

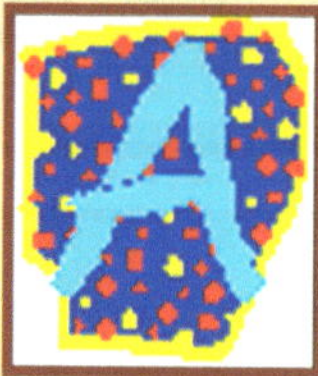

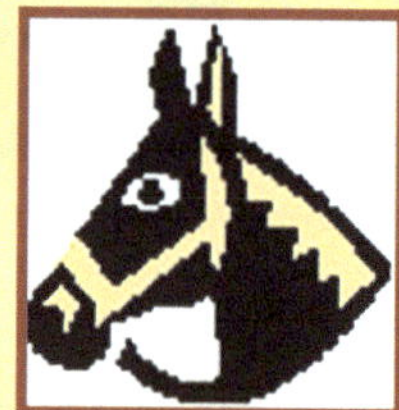

______ ______

E Y E
On
Colors

46. Which is your favorite color?

1 2 3 4 5 6 7

47. Tell me again. Which is your favorite color?

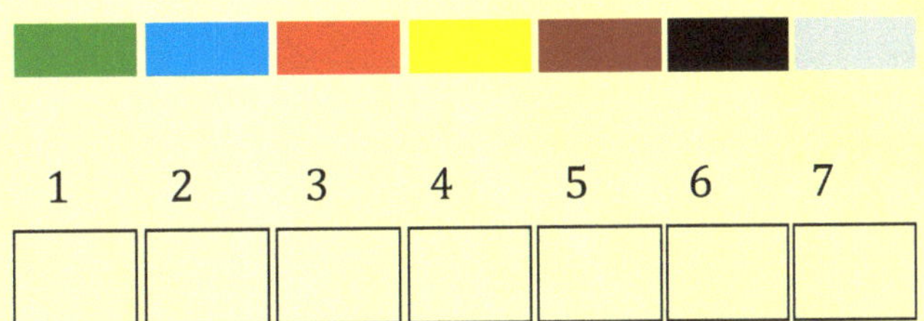

48. Place the yellow card on the pink card
Place the black card on the brown card
Place the blue card on the purple card
Place the orange card on the green card

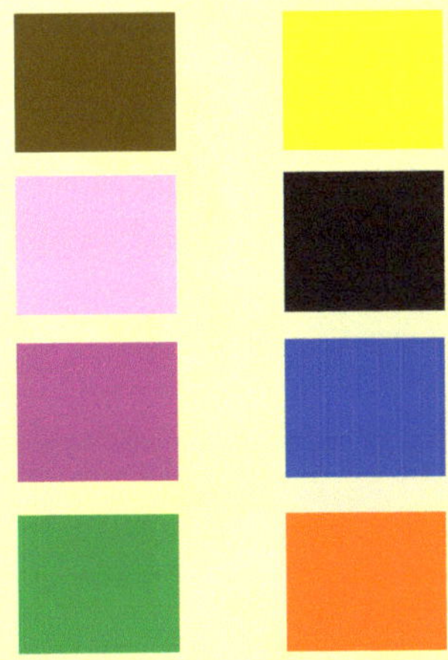

49. Now match the colors in order.

50. Put these pieces into the box.

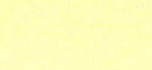

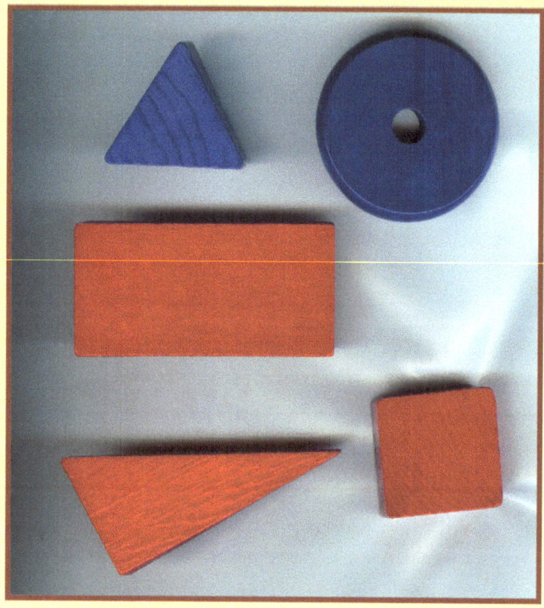

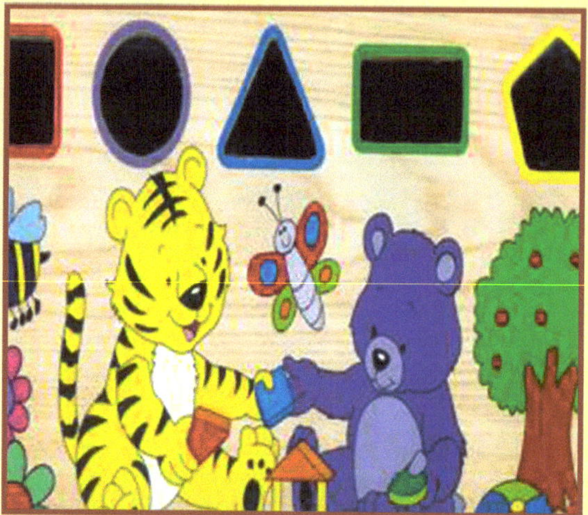

51. Use these pieces to put together the puzzle.

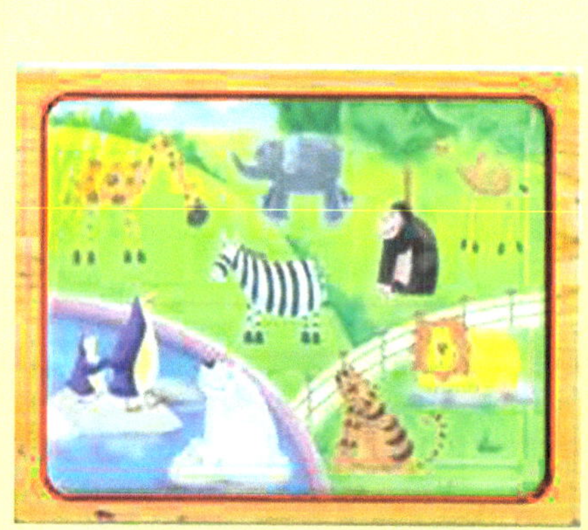

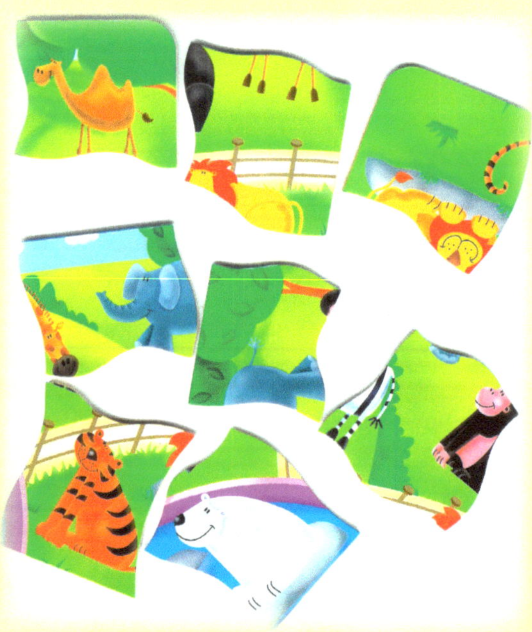

COMMENTS:

____

____

____

____

WORD POWER

52. An airplane flies in the ______________________________.

53. A bicycle has ______________________________wheels.

54. Fish swim in the______________________________.

55. My mommy cooks______________________________.

56. My mommy bakes______________________________.

57. Birds fly in the______________________________.

58. My daddy works in ______________________________.

59. I live at______________________________.

60. What is a telephone?______________________________.

61. Do you know your telephone number? Y N

62. What is it? ( )______/______/______

63. If someone gets hurt, you call______________________________.

64. Do you go to school? Y N

65. Do you want to go to school? Y N

66. Why? ______________________________

67. When do you go to sleep? ______________________________

68. When do you wake up? ______________________________

69. Do you go to the toilet? Y N Why?______________________________

70. Did you eat breakfast? Y N

71. What did you eat?______________________________

72. Do you cry sometimes? Y N

73. Why do you cry? ______________________________

74. Do you have friends? Y N

75. Who is your best friend? ______________________________

DRAWING ANALYSIS

76. Draw the things you see in the sky

77. Draw the things on earth

78. Color a rainbow

79. Draw a picture of your favorite pet or animal.

80. Now, draw a picture of you.

81. Draw a picture of your house.

82. Now draw a picture of your whole family.

83. Use the dots to draw a picture of a person, animal, and object.

84. Look at the dots and identify at least four images. Trace the images you see.

85. Draw a tree.

86. Insert eyes and a mouth between the branches.

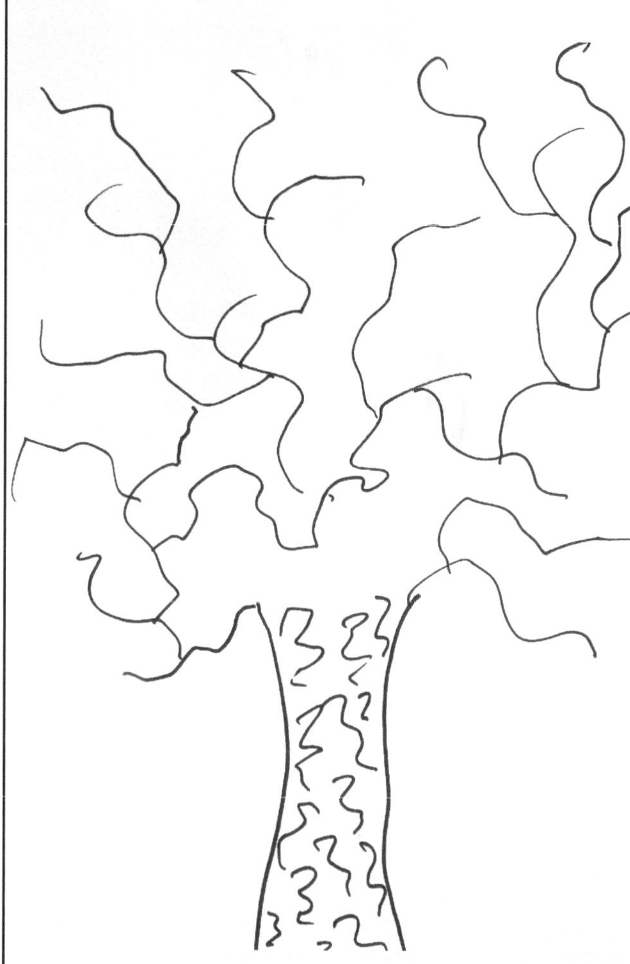

87. Specify all the images you see on the tree.

1____________________________

2____________________________

3____________________________

4____________________________

5____________________________

6____________________________

7____________________________

8____________________________

9____________________________

10____________________________

11____________________________

12____________________________

88. Draw two eyes in each box

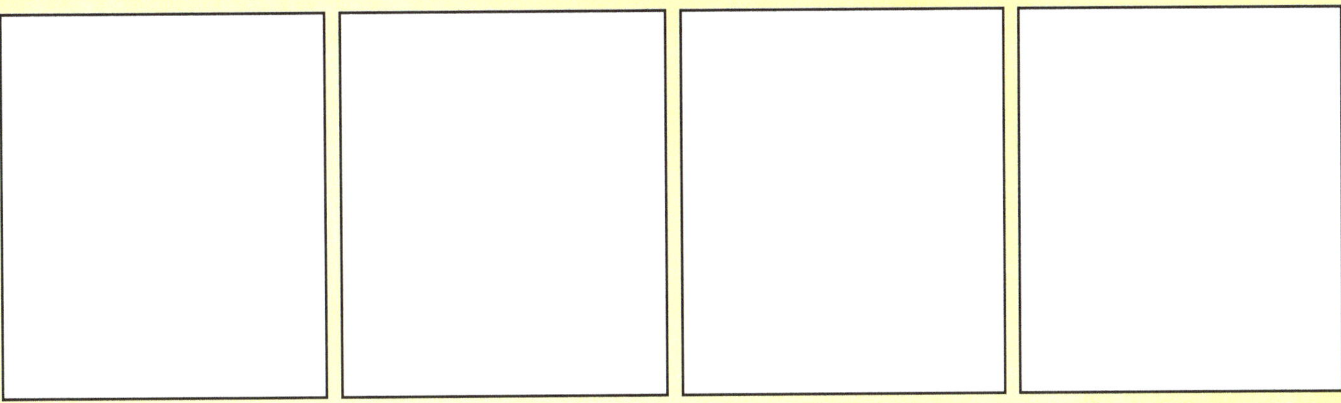

89.

1
Draw eyes in this image

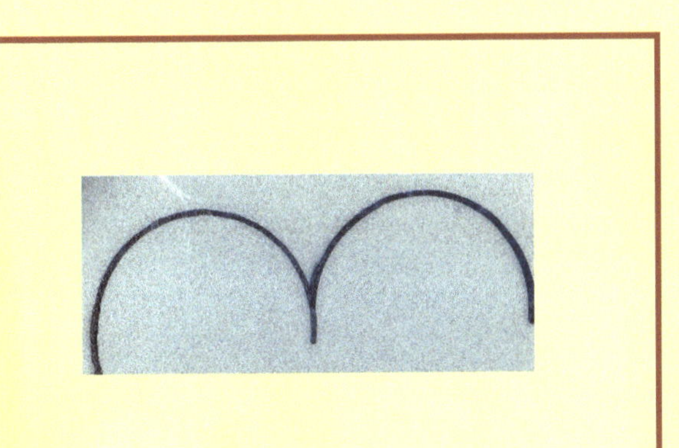

2
Draw eyes, a nose, and a mouth

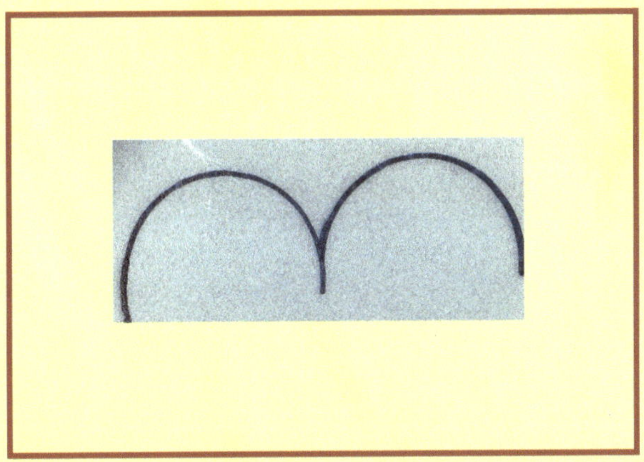

3
Draw eyes; a nose, mouth, and a head

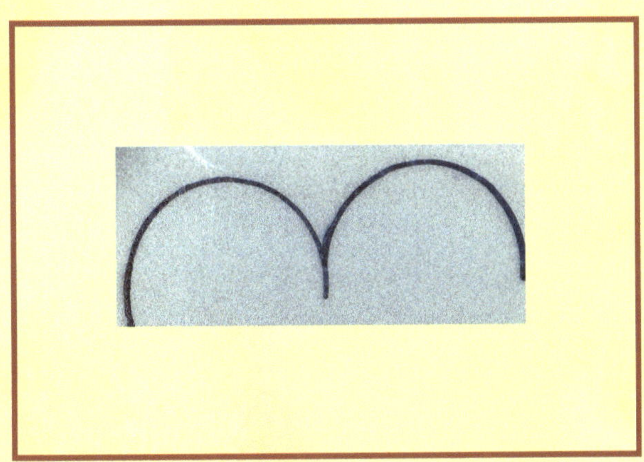

4
Complete the drawing

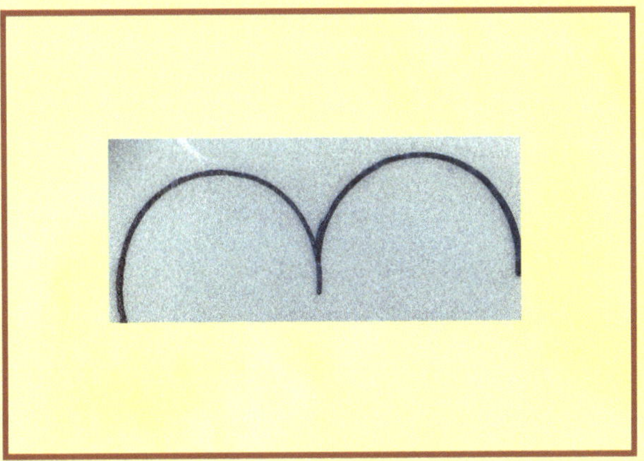

90 Scribble Analysis

Image 1

Image 4

Image 3

Image 2

---

91 Lead energizer

Image 1

Image 4

Image 3

Image 2

92 REVERSE IMAGE ANALYSIS

Black and white

93 REVERSE IMAGE ANALYSIS

Color

DATE___/___/___

NAME________________________________AGE__ GENDER M____ F____

IMAGE ONE

IMAGE FOUR

IMAGE THREE

IMAGE TWO

DUPLICATE

IMAGE ONE

IMAGE FOUR

IMAGE THREE

IMAGE TWO

CHILD'S WELFARE QUESTIONNAIR

PERSONAL

1. I like to be alone in my room. (T) (F)
2. I sleep with my mommy or with my daddy. (T) (F)
3. I love my family. (T) (F)
4. I hate my siblings. (T) (F)
5. I hate my daddy. (T) (F)
6. I love my mommy. (T) (F)
7. I think that my family loves me. (T) (F)
8. I am strong. (T) (F)
9. I like the way I look. (T) (F)
10. I am always happy. (T) (F)
11. I know how to play better than my brother does. (T) (F)
12. My sister/brother gets everything, and I have nothing. (T) (F)
13. My parents love me more than they love my siblings. (T) (F)
14. I like to listen to music. (T) (F)
15. I am always good. (T) (F)
16. I like to do things and go to places. (T) (F)
17. I love to go to school. (T) (F)
18. Everybody likes me in school. (T) (F)
19. I always like to play with my friends. (T) (F)
20. I like to play with my friends in their house only. (T) (F)
21. Sometimes I just want to stay home. (T) (F)
22. My mommy makes me go to places even when I am tired. (T) (F)
23. I am always bored. (T) (F)
24. I hate when other children come to my house. (T) (F)
25. I like to tease my pets. (T) (F)
26. I like hunting and fishing. (T) (F)
27. Child tends to wander away without permission from:

    (School) (Home) (Playground)

    (From a friend's house) (Backyard)

    (Mall) (Doctor's office) (other)

NUTRITION AND EATING HABITS:

Child's age ________ Religion ________

Height ________ Weight ________ Skin ________

28. Underweight. (T) (F)
29. Overweight. (T) (F)
30. Family thinks the child is too fat/skinny/normal. (T) (F)
31. Snacks more than eat regular meals. (T) (F)
32. Eats enough vegetables. (T) (F)
33. Exhibits tantrums if desired foods are restricted. (T) (F)
34. Eats at least three normal meals a day. (T) (F)
35. Prefers to drink sodas instead of water or juices. (T) (F)
36. Eats too fast (T) (F)
37. Eats too slow. (T) (F)
38. Eats fast food most of the time. (T) (F)
39. Refuses to eat in public. (T) (F)
40. Feeds him/herself independently. (T) (F)
41. Eats most of the meal near the TV. (T) (F)
42. Hides food and eats when no one sees. (T) (F)
43. Complains frequently about bellyaches. (T) (F)
44. Sticks his/her fingers down the throat to vomit. (T) (F)
45. Tends to overindulge. (T) (F)
46. Drinks with the food. (T) (F)
47. Parents are forcing food even when the child claims to be full. (T) (F)
48. Drinks coffee. (T) (F)
49. Likes to listen to music during meals. (T) (F)
50. Eats lots of salty foods. (T) (F)
51. A balanced diet is important for the child's good health. (T) (F)
52. Takes daily-prescribed vitamins. (T) (F)
53. Likes to help to cook. (T) (F)
54. Eats fried foods daily. (T) (F)
55. Decides what food to eat. (T) (F)
56. Parents believe that it is no one's business what a child eats. (T) (F)
57. Exhibits early signs for an eating disorder. (T) (F)
58. Blames parents for feeding him/her junk food. (T) (F)
59. Parents blame child for eating junk food. (T) (F)

This questionnaire is based on observations and conversations with parents and teachers. The core theme for this study is to monitor family nutritional habits and child's welfare.

LEISURE AND RECREATION

60. Doesn't mind talking to strangers. (T) (F)
61. Likes to start a conversation. (T) (F)
62. Feels comfortable talking on the phone. (T) (F)
63. Likes to play a musical instrument. (T) (F)
64. Likes to show off his/her talents to family and strangers. (T) (F)
65. Likes to take hikes with or without permission. (T) (F)
66. Likes to get attention in public. (T) (F)
67. Attends recreation activities at least twice a week. (T) (F)
68. Likes to listen to loud music. (T) (F)
69. Ignores parents' or strangers' complaints or comments. (T) (F)
70. Likes to read and listen to stories. (T) (F)
71. Demands to go out on freezing or hot days. (T) (F)
72. Enjoys playing in the park on nice days. (T) (F)
73. Was caught shoplifting or stealing. (T) (F)
74. Blames other children when he/she starts a fight during a game. (T) (F)
75. Tends to be friendly with troubled children. (T) (F)
76. Is often removed from a game due to bad behavior. (T) (F)
77. Has a favorite sport. (T) (F)
78. Likes swimming. (T) (F)
79. Hates to lose a game. (T) (F)
80. Winning makes him/her feel good. (T) (F)
81. Feels often cheated during games. (T) (F)
82. Gets angry when losing a game. (T) (F)
83. Likes to mess up the room and house. (T) (F)
84. Feels more comfortable staying at home. (T) (F)
85. Likes to travel. (T) (F)
86. Exhibits good behavior during family events. (T) (F)
87. Is happy to be with friends. (T) (F)
88. Is pleased with what he/she has. (T) (F)
89. Is happy with his/her gender. (T) (F)
90. Wishes to be of the opposite sex. (T) (F)

GROOMING AND HYGIENE

91. Brushes teeth at least once a day. (T) (F)
92. Showers daily. (T) (F)
93. Refuses to cut or brush hair. (T) (F)
94. Changes underwear daily. (T) (F)
95. Always dresses neatly. (T) (F)
96. Is conscious about his/her looks. (T) (F)
97. Hates his/her looks. (T) (F)
98. Feels that no one cares about his/her looks. (T) (F)
99. It makes me feel good when people praise my looks. (T) (F)
100. Hates to get dressed. (T) (F)
101. Puts up daily fights of what clothes to wear. (T) (F)
102. Is too lazy to get out of bed. (T) (F)
103. Shoes are always polished. (T) (F)
104. The clothes are wrinkled most of the time. (T) (F)
105. Feels comfortable the way he/she looks. (T) (F)
106. Cares when children comment about the way he/she dresses. (T) (F)
107. Cries when friends tell him/her to wipe his/her nose. (T) (F)
108. Everyone looks good. I am the only ugly one. (T) (F)
109. Every one likes the way I look. (T) (F)
110. People lie when they say, "You are looking good." (T) (F)
111. I don't care how I look. (T) (F)
112. Child's clothes are stained most of the time. (T) (F)
113. No one can tell when my shirt is stained. (T) (F)
114. Child smells from urine. (T) (F)
115. Toilet trained. Ages 2-5 (T) (F)
116. Still wets at night. (T) (F)
117. Nose is always running. (T) (F)
118. Refuses to wipe nose. (T) (F)
119. Wears shoes without stockings. (T) (F)
120. Shoes are worn out. (T) (F)
121. Legs and arms are often bruised or scratched. (T) (F)
122. Likes to wear a costume on Halloween/Purim. (T) (F)

PHYSICAL HEALTH

123. Is always sick. (T) (F)

124. Is afraid to sleep. (T) (F)

125. Sleeps with parents most of the time. (T) (F)

126. Doctors don't know what's wrong with him/her. (T) (F)

127. Parents and teachers are concerned for his/her health. (T) (F)

128. Likes to pretend to be sick to get attention. (T) (F)

129. Hates to get out of bed because he/she feels too tired. (T) (F)

130. Gets up early even when tired. (T) (F)

131. Wakes up more than one time at night to go to the bathroom. (T) (F)

132. Gets frequent headaches at night (T) (F)

133. Dreams a lot. (T) (F)

134. Often gets short of breath. (T) (F)

135. Has frequent nightmares. (T) (F)

136. Complains about aches and pains. (T) (F)

137. Parent feeds over the counter pain medications to calm child down. (T) (F)

138. Parent visits pediatrician frequently for any emotional or physical problem. (T) (F)

139. Parent fabricates an illness to get a quicker appointment to a pediatrician. (T) (F)

140. Parent threatens child to take him/her to the hospital if child does not behave. (T) (F)

141. Parent consults with pediatrician about what medications to give. (T) (F)

142. Parent ignores child's complaints about pain or ill feelings. (T) (F)

143. People get involved when the child is sick. (T) (F)

144. Prescribed drugs never help. (T) (F)

145. Parent uses own judgment as to how much medication to give the child. (T) (F)

146. Name all prescribed and over-the-counter drugs and dosages your child is taking.

____
____
____
____

147. What do doctors think is wrong with your child?

____
____
____
____

148. What do you think is wrong with your child?

____
____

149. Please check all items that relate to your child's health conditions.

Asthma_Blood disorders_ Cancer_ ADD_ Constipation_ADHD_Emotional_Diabetes_ Diarrhea__Pneumonia__Dizziness and fainting spells_ Diabetes_Edema_Fatigue_ Inherited diseases_ Mental retardation_Gastritis_ Hearing loss_ Heart condition _ HIV_ Hypertension__Anemia__Injuries__Kidney disease_ Liver disease_ Headaches_ Obesity_ Skin disease_ Sleep disorders _ Frequent urinary tract infections_ Vision impairment_ Hearing loss_Physical disability_Bruises easily_Bleeds frequently_

Others__________________________________

MENTAL HEALTH

150. Gets gloomy for no reason. (T) (F)
151. Feels bored and lonely even when there are children with him/her. (T) (F)
152. Daydreams a lot and cries. (T) (F)
153. Expresses wishes to die. (T) (F)
154. Gets angry for no reason. (T) (F)
155. Doesn't feel like doing anything. (T) (F)
156. Feels good to wake up every morning. (T) (F)
157. Enjoys life. (T) (F)
158. Blames him/herself for family issues. (T) (F)
159. Cries when parents go to work. (T) (F)
160. Refuses to go to play school. (T) (F)
161. Feels loved. (T) (F)
162. Hates when people tell him/her what to do. (T) (F)
163. Hates other children. (T) (F)
164. Punches and kicks when angry. (T) (F)
165. Throws objects, kicks, hits, screams, and curses when angry. (T) (F)
166. When another child touches his/her toy, child curses, bites, and hits. (T) (F)
167. Officials have no right to tell me how to raise my child. (T) (F)
168.When someone gives me advise, I smile and say thank you. (T) (F)

better. (T) (F)

169. Family believes in God. (T) (F)
170. Parent relies on miracles. (T) (F)
171. Parent is afraid of death. (T) (F)
172. Child knows about heaven and hell. (T) (F)
173. Parent believes that there is justice in this world. (T) (F)
174. Family turns to God in times of despair. (T) (F)
175. No one loves me, and no one cares about me. (T) (F)
176. Parents never thank God enough when the child feels better. (T) (F)
177. Child seems optimistic. (T) (F)
178. An illness is part of nature, and God should never be blamed. (T) (F)
179. People get sick at all ages. (T) (F)
180. There are sicker people than your child. (T) (F)
181. Does not care about other people's anguish. (T) (F)
182. Faith in God is important. (T) (F)
183. No one cares how I feel. (T) (F)

PSYCHOSOCIAL

184. Prefers to play alone. (T) (F)
185. Likes to eat in public. (T) (F)
186. Too shy to speak in public. (T) (F)
187. Self conscious. (T) (F)
188. Hates to look into the mirror. (T) (F)
189. Everyone is stupid. (T) (F)
190. Knows better than others. (T) (F)
191. Blames others for his/her faults. (T) (F)
192. Extremely sensitive to smell. (T) (F)
193. Extremely sensitive to noise. (T) (F)
194. Hates crowds. (T) (F)
195. Tends to argue with peers. (T) (F)
196. Seeks attention in public. (T) (F)
197. Cheats during games. (T) (F)
198. Tends to criticize. (T) (F)
199. Likes to push. (T) (F)
200. Takes revenge when someone pushes him/her accidentally. (T) (F)
201. Bullies other children. (T) (F)
202. Pinches, bites, and hits for no specific reason. (T) (F)
203. Demonstrates cruelty to animals. (T) (F)
204. Feels socially accepted. (T) (F)
205. Does not hesitate to speak to strangers. (T) (F)
206. More hyperactive in public than at home (T) (F)
207. Gets annoyed when parent speaks to a friend. (T) (F)
208. Nags when parent has company. (T) (F)
209. Gets often hurt. (T) (F)
210. Cries for attention. (T) (F)
211. Calls himself/herself names for attention. (T) (F)
212. Uses negative words too often. (T) (F)

1__________32__________

2__________33__________

3__________34__________

4__________35__________

5__________36__________

6__________37__________

7__________38__________

8__________39__________

9__________40__________

10__________41__________

11__________42__________

12__________43__________

13__________44__________

14__________45__________

15__________46__________

16__________47__________

17__________48__________

18__________49__________

19__________50__________

20__________51__________

21__________52__________

22__________53__________

23__________54__________

24__________55__________

25__________56__________

26__________57__________

27__________58__________

28__________59__________

29__________60__________

30__________61__________

31__________62__________

63__________94__________

64__________95__________

65__________96__________

66__________97__________

67__________98__________

68__________99__________

69__________100__________

70__________101__________

71__________102__________

72__________103__________

73__________104__________

74__________105__________

75__________106__________

76__________107__________

77__________108__________

78__________109__________

79 __________ 110__________

80__________111__________

82__________113__________

83 __________ 114__________

84__________115__________

85__________116__________

86__________117__________

87 __________ 118__________

88__________119__________

89__________120__________

90__________121__________

91 __________ 122__________

92__________123__________

93__________124__________

125________155__________
126________156__________
127________157__________
128________158__________
129________159__________
130________160__________
131________161__________
132________162__________
133________163__________
134________164__________
135________165__________
136________166__________
137________167__________
138________168__________
139________169__________
140________170__________
141________171__________
142________172__________
143________173__________
144________174__________
145________175__________
146________176__________
147________177__________
148________178__________
149________179__________
150________180__________
151________181__________
152________182__________
153________183__________
154________184__________

185__________
186__________
187__________
188__________
189__________
190__________
191__________
192__________
193__________
194__________
195__________
196__________
197__________
198__________
199__________
200__________
201__________
202__________
203__________
204__________
205__________
206__________
207__________
208__________
209__________
210__________
211__________
212__________

STANDARD SCORES FOR EARLY CHILDHOOD GEDDI APTITUDE TEST

TODAY'S DATE____/____/____

Name:____________________ D.O.B.______/______/______ S.S.#______-______-______
Address:____

Telephone: (_____)______/________Cell: (_____)______/________
E-mail____

SUBJECT	QUANTITY	MAXIMUM	TOTAL (T)	TOTAL (F)	SCORE	RATIO
PERSONAL:	24	235	14 (T)	10 (F) =	14/10 =	1.4
PSYCHOSOCIAL:	29	235	2 (T)	27 (F) =	2/27 =	0.07
NUTRITION:	32	235	8 (T)	24 (F) =	8/24 =	0.33
LEISURE AND REC:	32	235	15 (T)	17 (F) =	15/17 =	0.88
HYGIENE:	32	235	12 (T)	20 (F) =	12/20 =	0. 6
PHYSICAL HEALTH:	27	235	3 (T)	24 (F) =	3/24 =	0.125
MENTAL HEALTH	37	235	12 (T)	25 (F) =	12/25 =	0.48
SPIRITUALITY	20	235	4 (T)	16 (F) =	4/16 =	0.25

$\frac{\text{70 True answers}}{\text{166 False answers}} = 0.42$ RATIO OF $\frac{70}{166} = 0.42$ or 42%

MENTAL HEALTH

These scores are based on a study conducted on a group of "normal," with delayed development, mental retardation, and physical disabilities.

The results are determined by the amount of children tested for this exam. In this case, the average group scored 47 %

THE EMOTIONALLY CHALLENGED SCORED

3.0+1.5+2+1.5+1.5+1.5+3.0+0.55 =14.55

THE MENTALLY CHALLENGED SCORED

5+5+6+3+4+4+5+0.2 =32.2

THE PHYSICALLY DISABLED SCORED

4.0+3.0+3.0+5.0+5.0+3.0+6.0++0.6 =2 9.6

4.55+.19+.94+.6+. 35+. 25+1.86+0.64 =6.08

THE AVERAGE "NORMAL" GROUP SCORED

1.4+0.07+0.33+0.88+0.6+0.125+0.48+0.25=4.135

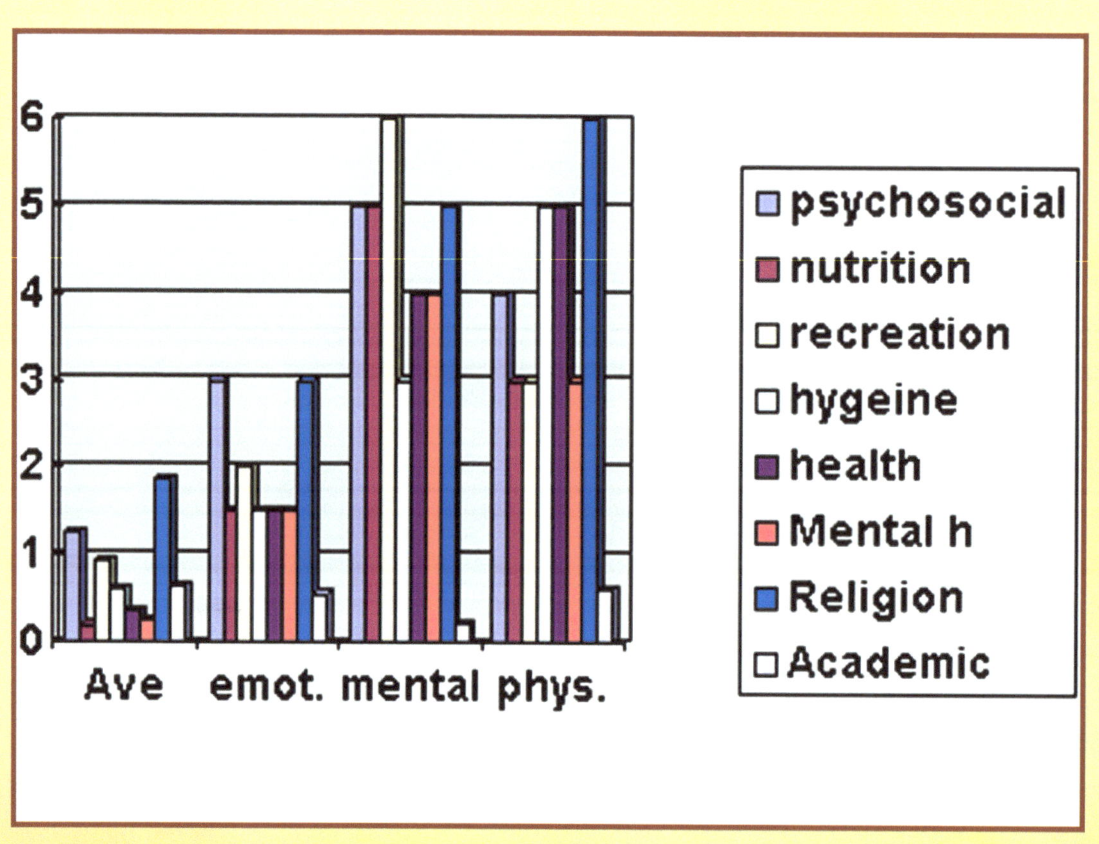

Please take note that the following pages hold the GEDDI examinations for children and adults.

OBJECTIVES FOR CHILDREN AND ADULTS:

1. Changing dreams and visions into art.
2. Understanding visions and dreams.
3. Expanding artistic skills.
4. Child development.
5. Psychoanalysis.
6. Maximize academic potentials.
7. Employment interrogation.
8. Legal examination.
9. To understand the meaning and the mechanical system of all energies.
10. To introduce the power of the eye and mind.

EYE INTELLIGENCE PROFILING

For children and adults

TODAY'S DATE____/____/__________
NAME: ____________________________
D. O. B.: ________/_______/_________
SEX: (M) (F)
TEL:( )________________________
ADDRESS:___________________________
SCHOOL:____________________________

(EIP GOALS)
L_____ 6______L
L______5______L
L____4____ L
L___3___ L
L__2__ L
L_1_L

ADVANCED LEVEL
1____2____3____4____5___6___

______________________	11	D
______________________	10	E
HS____________________	9	S
______________________	8	I
______________________	7	R
JH ___________________	6	E
______________________	5	D
______________________	4	
______________________	3	G
______________________	2	R
EL____________________	1	A
KG____________________	0	D
0___1___2___3___4___5___6___		E

LEVEL OF ACHIEVEMENT

COMMENTS: ________________
____
____
____
____
____
____
____
____
____
____
____

SCORE CHART

ITEM 1	ITEM 2	ITEM 3	ITEM 4	ITEM 5	ITEM 6	STANDARD POINT

MAP	=	MAXIMUM ACHIEVEMENT	150 -160
AP	=	ADVANCED POINT	72 -150
IP	=	INTERMEDIATE POINT	50 - 72
AP	=	AVERAGE POINT	32 - 50
BAV	=	BELOW AVERAGE	18 - 32
ALP	=	ABOVE LOWEST POINT	8 - 18
LP	=	LOWEST POINT	2 - 8

MENU FOR GEDDI STANDARDIZED TEST

1	2	3	4	5	6
ACADEMIC	PSYCHOSOCIAL	MOTOR SKILLS	COGNITIVE	ARTS	VERBAL

1) TO ESTABLISH A MAXIMUM POINT VALUE SYSTEM

$\frac{\text{MAXIMUM SCORE 160}}{\text{ITEMS} \quad 6} = 26.6$ CHECK: MAP= 26.6X6=159.6 OR 160

2) TO ESTABLISH AN AVERAGE POINT VALUE SYSTEM

If the academic falls in the 80%, psychosocial 65%, motor skills 40% mental 50%, arts 25% and verbal skills in the 20%. Calculate 80+65+40+50+25+20=255

$\frac{255}{6 \text{ ITEMS}} = 42.5$ $\frac{42.5}{160} = 0.26$ OR 26%

3) TO ESTABLISH A MINIMUM POINT VALUE SYSTEM

If an average point value is 26%, a minimum point value should not be less than ten points below the average score. For instance 26-10= $\frac{16}{6 \text{ ITEMS}} = 2.67$

EXAMPLE:

WRITING SKILLS	5 POINTS
MATH	8 POINTS
VERBAL EXPRESSION	10 POINTS
READING	15 POINTS
PSYCHOSOCIAL	2 POINTS
EYE HAND COORDINATION	12 POINTS
TOTAL POINTS	52=8.6 6 ITEMS
AVERAGE POINT ACHIEVED	8.6

POINT=LIP 8.6 =0.053 0.053X8.6=0.4558=45.58 OR 46%
MP = 160

$\frac{\text{48 ITEMS}}{\text{244 TOTAL QUESTIONS}}$ = 0.196 points for each correct answer

MIPQ= $\frac{0.196}{160}$ =0.001225 0.001225 X 0.196=0.0002401 X 100%=0.02401 OR 2.4%

GEDDI APTITUDE TEST

TODAY'S DATE____/____/___

ACADEMIC

1__________ 25__________
2__________ 26__________
3__________ 27__________
4__________ 28__________
5__________ 29__________
6__________ 30__________
7__________ 31__________
8__________ 32__________
9__________ 33__________
10__________ 34__________
11__________ 35__________
12__________ 36__________
13__________ 37__________
14__________ 38__________
15__________ 39__________
16__________ 40__________
17__________ 41__________
18__________ 42__________
19__________ 43__________
20__________ 44__________
21__________ 45__________
22__________ 46__________
23__________ 47__________
24__________ 48__________

TOTAL SCORE________/48

1. What is your telephone number? ____________________

2. What is your home address? ____________________

____

3. What time is it now? ____________________

4. What is today's day and date? ____________________

5. How many minutes are there in one hour? ____________________

6. What time is noon? ____________________

7. How many hours are there in a day? ____________________

8. How many days are there in a week? ____________________

9. How many months are there in one year? ____________________

10. How many weeks are there in one year? ____________________

11. How many days are 48 hours? ____________________

12. Tell the months backwards in order beginning with December.

1__________ 7__________

2__________ 8__________

3__________ 9__________

4__________ 10__________

5__________ 11__________

6__________ 12__________

13. What month comes after May?____________________

14. What month comes before January? ____________________

15. October is which month of the year? ____________________

16. How many months are there from September to January? ____________________

17. What is the last month of the year? ____________________

18. What county do you live in? ____________________

19. What state do you live in? ____________________

20. If Isaac was born in May, and George was born in November of the same year, who is older, and by how many months?

____

____

21. Where is the capital of your state? ____________________

22. Where is the capital of the United States? ______________________________

23. Who is the current president of the U.S.A.? ____________________________

24. Who is the vise-president of the U.S.A.? ________________________________

25. Which is the highest court in America? _________________________________

26. How many states are there in the U.S.A.? _______________________________

27. What do a marker, pen, and pencil have in common? ___________________

28. What do the moon, stars, and sun have in common? ___________________

29. What do parents, rabbi/ priest, and teachers have in common? __________

____

30. What do whales, fish, and dolphins have in common? __________________

31. Name three living creatures that walk on two feet.

____

____

____

32. Which grows taller, a tree or a bush? ___________________________________

33. Name three things you do before you leave the house.

____

____

____

34. What are the differences among:

Farms____

Towns____

Cities____

Settlements____

Colonies____

Ranches____

35. What is the difference between a:

Horse and a donkey

____

Fruit and a vegetable

____

Boat and a raft

____

Boat and a plane

___

Hole and a crater

___

Star and the moon

___

36. Fill in the blank.

Hello! My name is ________and I live in a________ near a ________. Every morning, when the ________are still________, I like to stand near the________ ________and stare into the________and think about________ ________ and hope I could________ ________ ________. Day comes, and day________. Life is like a________. I hope for ________. When I snap out of my deep________, the ________ seems different. Another day has gone by. The air cools down, and ________falls on the________. There is ________again. I cannot________; so I stand near the________and admire the beauty of ________. I am happy with what ________but sad when I think about________. I miss the times when ________ and I would visit our beautiful________. Now, all I can feel is a ________in my life. If I could only________ ________chance, and tell________ what I really think, I would be the ________ ________person on earth. I am afraid of the________. If anyone could just ________ ________to what I have to ________, maybe I could convince the________ how________I am. Now I am looking forward to a new________and learn how to admire the brightness of________. Life is not as ________ as I think.

VOCABULARY

37. Match the following words:

    __Bright------------------------- A__mean

    __Brave--------------------------B__shelter

    __Gritty--------------------------C__fuming

    __Courage-----------------------D__Stingy

    __Protection--------------------E__brilliant

    __Furious------------------------F__grainy

Eye on Numbers

38. 6+7 =__________
39. 72-35 =__________
40. 9+1.23+25.368+122.001+0.12=________
41. $5\overline{)15}$ 42. $11\overline{)33}$

43. $33\overline{)69}$ 44. $12\overline{)128}$

45. 3X4 =__________
46. 9X6 =__________
47. 26X32 =__________
48. 163X2 =__________
49. 94X194 =__________
50. 1.33X12 =__________
51. 55X25.7 =__________
52. $\frac{1}{6}+\frac{5}{6}$ =__________
53. $\frac{5}{9}-\frac{8}{9}$ =__________
54. $\frac{3}{9}$ X $\frac{6}{12}$ =__________
55. $\frac{3}{16}-\frac{6}{32}$ =__________
56. 5X=40
    X=______________
57. 8X=64
    X=______________
58. $\frac{3}{12}$ X $\frac{6}{12}$ =__________
59. $\frac{3}{16}-\frac{6}{16}$ =__________

60. Organize the numbers from the least to the highest number.

16 32 20 21 19 36

__ __ __ __ __ __

SOLVE FOR X

61. 5X=20
    X=______
62. 8X+X+3X =____________
63. X+X+2X+8X=__________
64. X+9=50 50-X=9 77:X=11
    X=___ X=___ X=___
65. 15X17=X 99+X=999
    X=____ X=____
66. 100-X=75 X=________
67. Rewrite the numbers from the highest to the lowest
    52 179 43 152 409 88 94 61 629
    __ __ __ __ __ __ __ __ __
68. FILL IN A (+) OR A (-)

19___96___102___60____20___17___34
___36___963___593___349___126___17____

69. Solve the following problems.

Jonathan's mother gave him $11.97 for lunch. He bought one cupcake for .75 cents, a small orange juice for $1.99, and potato chips for .60 cents.

How much money did Jonathan spend?

____

How much change did he get back?

____

70. Sue went on a round trip to and from the Bahamas. She traveled 20 miles from her home to the boat, and 60 miles from the boat to the Bahamas.

How many miles did Sue travel one way?

____

How many miles did she travel in total?

____

71. A train and a racing car left from Chicago going to Maryland at the same time. If the distance from Chicago to Maryland is 800 miles, and the train was moving 500 miles per hour, how many hours did it take for the train to get to its destination?______________

How many hours did it take for the racing car to get to Maryland if a person drove 120 miles per hour? ____________

How many hours faster did the train arrive?_____________

72. SOLVE THE PUZZLES

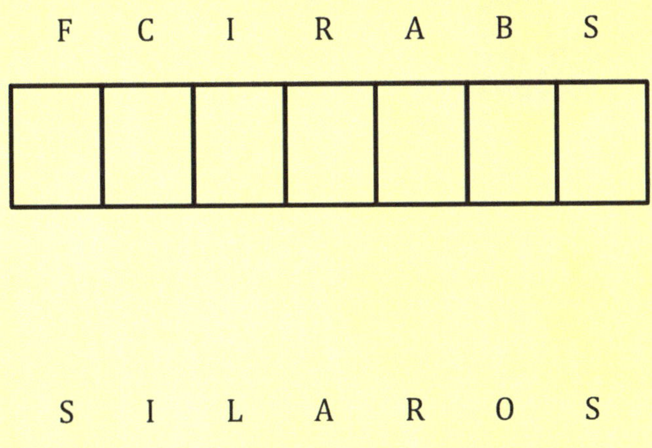

S I L A R O S

E YE
ON
SHAPES

73. Circle two items that have nothing in common.

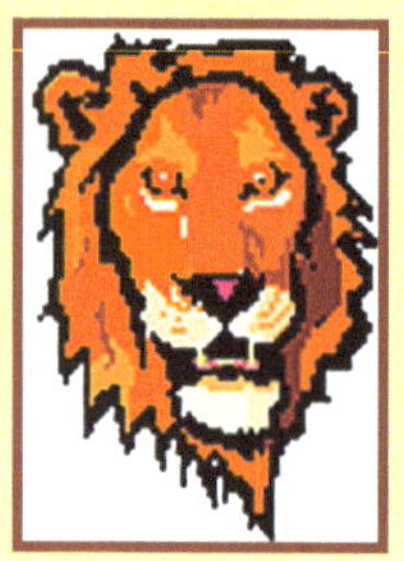
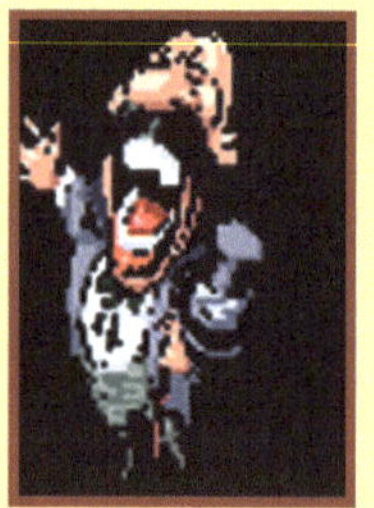
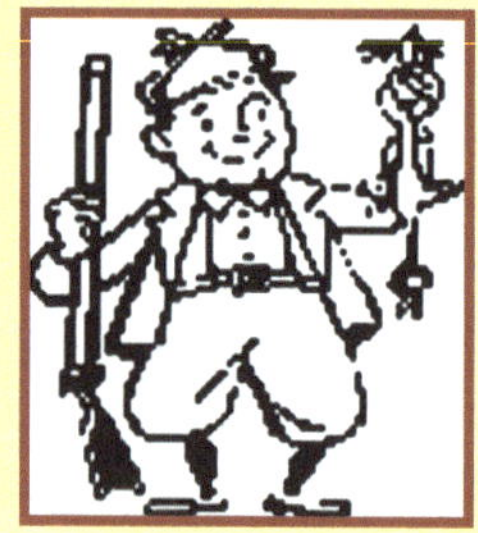
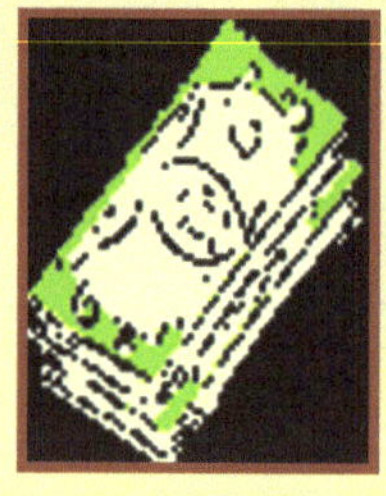
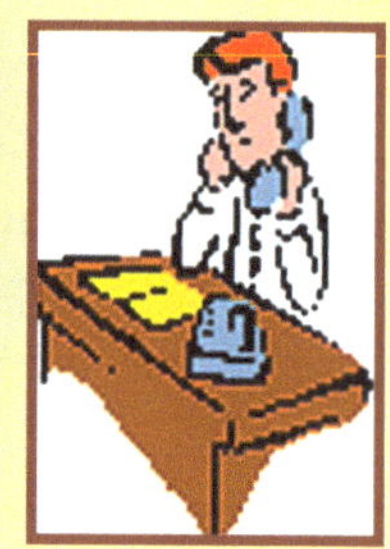
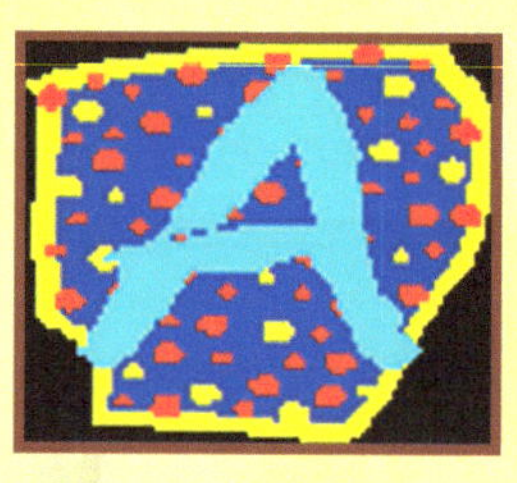

74. Name each shape below.

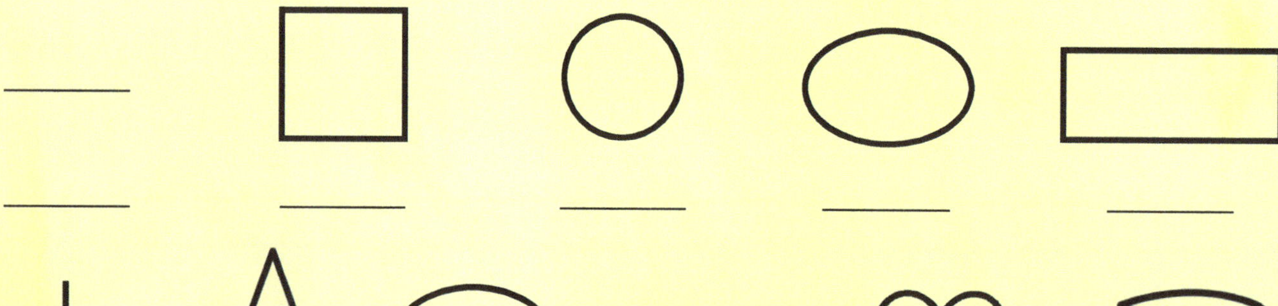

E Y E
On
Colors

75. Write the numbers under the colored boxes in order from the least to your most favorite color.

1	2	3	4	5	6	7

76. Memorize the colors above from your least to most favorite colors, and color the lines below in your new order.

1	2	3	4	5	6	7

77. In a five-sentence paragraph write about your favorite color, and what the color means to you.

____

____

____

____

____

PSYCHOSOCIAL

78__________	95__________
79__________	96__________
80__________	97__________
81__________	98__________
82__________	99__________
83__________	100__________
84__________	101__________
85__________	102__________
86__________	103__________
87__________	104__________
88__________	105__________
89__________	106__________
90__________	107__________
91__________	108__________
92__________	109__________
93__________	110__________
94__________	111__________

$$\frac{\text{32 QUESTIONS}}{\text{290 TOTAL QUESTIONS}} = 0.11 \text{ points}$$

$$\frac{\text{290 TOTAL QUESTIONS}}{160} = 1.81 = \text{MIPQ}$$

0.11X1.81=0.199X100%=19.9 OR 20%

If 17 answers are True and
15 answers are False
The "ratio" would be 17/15
or 1.13x20=22.6%

78. I like to be alone. (T) (F)

79. I feel lonely even when I am surrounded with people. (T) (F)

80. I hate my family. (T) (F)

81. I hate my siblings. (T) (F)

82. I hate my father. (T) (F)

83. I love my mother. (T) (F)

84. My family does not care about me. (T) (F)

85. I am a loser. (T) (F)

86. I hate myself. (T) (F)

87. I am always happy. (T) (F)

88. I know some things better than other people do. (T) (F)

89. My friends have everything they want, and I have nothing. (T) (F)

90. My parents love me more than they love my siblings. (T) (F)

91. I wish I were never born. (T) (F)

92. Life is always good. (T) (F)

93. I keep busy when I am alone. (T) (F)

94. I love to go to school. (T) (F)

95. I am the most popular student. (T) (F)

96. At work, I always work the hardest. (T) (F)

97. I like to visit friends. (T) (F)

98. Sometimes I feel that life is worthless. (T) (F)

99. I fit in to every group. (T) (F)

100. Life goes too slow for me. (T) (F)

101. I have enough family support. (T) (F)

102. I hate children. (T) (F)

103. I like to tease and torture animals. (T) (F)

104. I like hunting. (T) (F)

105. I often disappear from home. (T) (F)

106. I drink an alcoholic beverage more than one cup a day. (T) (F)

107. I smoke more than one box of cigarettes a day. (T) (F)

108. I tend to break the law. (T) (F)

109. I have shoplifted more than once. (T) (F)

NUTRITION AND EATING HABITS	
110__________	124__________
111__________	125__________
112__________	126__________
113__________	127__________
114__________	128__________
115__________	129__________
116__________	130__________
117__________	131__________
118__________	132 __________
119__________	133__________
120__________	134__________
121__________	135__________
122__________	136__________
123__________	137__________
138__________	140__________
139__________	141__________

$$\frac{\text{32 QUESTIONS}}{\text{290 TOTAL QUESTIONS}} = 0.11 \text{ points}$$

$$\frac{\text{290 TOTAL QUESTIONS}}{160} = 1.81 = \text{MIPQ}$$

0.11X1.81=0.2079X100%=20.79 OR 21%

If 17 answers are True and
15 answers are False
The "ratio" would be 17/15
or 1.13x19.83=(22.41)%

---

110. I hate to be skinny. (T) (F)

111. I feel too fat. (T) (F)

112. People tell me that I am too fat. (T) (F)

113. Ice cream is my favorite food. (T) (F)

114. Green vegetables are good for me. (T) (F)

115. I like candy more than fruits. (T) (F)

116. I must eat cake for desert. (T) (F)

117. I eat at least three meals a day. (T) (F)

118. I prefer to eat out. (T) (F)

119. I hate to eat in public. (T) (F)

120. I like to eat alone. (T) (F)

121. I eat near the TV or at the computer. (T) (F)

122. I like to eat when no one sees what I eat. (T) (F)

123. I regret eating after meals. (T) (F)

124. I put my fingers down my throat to vomit after meals. (T) (F)

125. Sometimes I watch what I eat, and other times I overindulge. (T) (F)

126. I drink with the food. (T) (F)

127. I hate water. I prefer to drink soda. (T) (F)

128. I like to smoke and drink coffee after meals. (T) (F)

129. I like to listen to music during meals. (T) (F)

130. I eat lots of salty foods. (T) (F)

131. A balanced diet is important for good health. (T) (F)

132. I am taking daily vitamins. (T) (F)

133. I like to cook. (T) (F)

134. Fried foods are delicious and very healthy. (T) (F)

135. I hate when people decide what's good for me. (T) (F)

136. It is no one's business if I am anorexic or bulimic. (T) (F)

137. I have an eating disorder. (T) (F)

138. I blame my parents or spouse for my eating disorder. (T) (F)

139. I am responsible for my own actions. (T) (F)

LEISURE AND RECREATION

140________	148________	156________	164________
141________	149________	157________	165________
142________	150________	158________	166________
143________	151________	159________	167________
144________	152________	160________	168________
145________	153________	161________	169________
146________	154________	162________	170________
147________	155________	163________	171________

$$\frac{\text{32 QUESTIONS}}{\text{290 TOTAL QUESTIONS}} = 0.11 \text{ points}$$

$$\frac{\text{290 TOTAL QUESTIONS}}{160} = 1.81 = \text{MIPQ}$$

0.11X1.81=0.2079X100%=20.79 OR 21%

If 17 answers are True and
15 answers are False
The "ratio" would be 17/15
or 1.13x19.83=(22.41)%

140. I share my musical talents with others. (T) (F)

141. I like to hitchhike. (T) (F)

142. I like to play loud music. (T) (F)

143. I don't care about people's complaints. (T) (F)

144. I like to read. (T) (F)

145. I go to the park on nice days. (T) (F)

146. Shopping is my best activity. (T) (F)

147. I often shoplift because I cannot control this temptation. (T) (F)

148. I like to get attention in public. (T) (F)

149. I go to a health club at least twice a week. (T) (F)

150. I often feel cheated during table games. (T) (F)

151. I belong to a group of people who violate the law. (T) (F)

152. Hanging out with criminals is cool. (T) (F)

153. I often cheat on my partner/friend. (T) (F)

154. I play tennis. (T) (F)

155. Swimming is the best sport. (T) (F)

156. I hate to lose a game. (T) (F)

157. Winning makes me feel good. (T) (F)

158. Do you gamble? (T) (F)

159. I tend to get angry when I lose a game. (T) (F)

160. I often like to rearrange the house. (T) (F)

161. I feel comfortable at home. (T) (F)

162. I love to travel to other states and countries. (T) (F)

163. I am happy with my partner/friend. (T) (F)

164. I am pleased with my sex life. (T) (F)

165. I don't mind talking to strangers. (T) (F)

166. I am happy with my gender. (T) (F)

167. I wish I would be of the opposite sex. (T) (F)

168. I prefer talking on the phone than facing people. (T) (F)

169. I play a musical instrument. (T) (F)

170. I believe that whatever God gives is for the best. (T) (F)

171. I like to start a conversation. (T) (F)

GROOMING AND HYGIENE

173.________	181.________	189________	197________
174.________	182.________	190________	198________
175.________	183________	191________	199________
176.________	184________	192________	200________
177________	185________	193________	201________
178.________	186________	194________	202________
179.________	187________	195________	203________
180.________	188________	196________	204________

$$\frac{\text{32 QUESTIONS}}{\text{290 TOTAL QUESTIONS}} = 0.11 \text{ points}$$

$$\frac{\text{290 TOTAL QUESTIONS}}{160} = 1.81 = \text{MIPQ}$$

0.11X1.81=0.2079X100%=20.79 OR 21%

If <u>17</u> answers are True and
15 answers are False
The "ratio" would be 17/15 or 1.13x19.83=(22.41)%

172. I brush my teeth at least once a day. (T) (F)

173. I shower daily. (T) (F)

174. I never cut or style my hair. (T) (F)

175. It is not necessary to change underwear daily. (T) (F)

176. It is not necessary to dress up at home. (T) (F)

177. I am too ugly. Makeup will not improve my looks. (T) (F)

178. There is nothing I can do for my pimples. (T) (F)

179. No one even cares how I look. (T) (F)

180. A bit of cologne and some hand cream makes me feel good. (T) (F)

181. I would rather throw away my clothes than fix them. (T) (F)

182. When I dress nicely, I feel attractive. (T) (F)

183. I am too lazy to wash laundry. (T) (F)

184. No one polishes shoes anymore. (T) (F)

185. I never iron clothes even when they are wrinkled. (T) (F)

186. I am good looking, and I don't have to impress others. (T) (F)

187. I get offended when people tell me that my teeth are yellow. (T) (F)

188. I don't think that I deserve to look good. (T) (F)

189. Everyone looks good. I am the only ugly one. (T) (F)

190. People tell me that I look neat and well groomed. (T) (F)

191. People lie when they say, "You are looking good." (T) (F)

192. I care how I look. (T) (F)

193. I like to dress in solid colors. (T) (F)

194. I like to wear clothes with prints. (T) (F)

195. I never put attention for the way I dress as long as my clothes are clean. (T) (F)

196. No one can tell when my shirt is stained. (T) (F)

197. I am responsible for the way I dress and groom. (T) (F)

198. I never got a manicure or pedicure. (T) (F)

199. I don't go to beauty salons because of contagious diseases. (T) (F)

200. I hate the way street girls dress. (T) (F)

201. Cowboys look cool. (T) (F)

202. Business people look very attractive. (T) (F)

203. It is not necessary to change looks for special events. (T) (F)

PHYSICAL HEALTH	
205______	215______
206______	216______
207______	217______
208______	218______
209______	219______
210______	220______
211______	221______
212______	222______
213______	223______
214______	224______

$$\frac{\text{32 QUESTIONS}}{\text{290 TOTAL QUESTIONS}} = 0.11 \text{ points}$$

$$\frac{\text{290 TOTAL QUESTIONS}}{160} = 1.81 = \text{MIPQ}$$

0.11X1.81=0.2079X100%=20.79 OR 21%

If 17 answers are True and
15 answers are False
The "ratio" would be 17/15
or 1.13x19.83=(22.41)%

204. I am always sick. (T) (F)

205. I am afraid to die. (T) (F)

206. I wish to die. (T) (F)

207. Doctors don't know what's wrong with me. (T) (F)

208. I am always preoccupied with my health. (T) (F)

209. I like to pretend to be sick to get attention. (T) (F)

210. I hate to get out of bed because I am tired. (T) (F)

211. I can get up early even when I feel tired. (T) (F)

212. I wake up more than one time at night to go to the bathroom. (T) (F)

213. I get frequent headaches at night. (T) (F)

214. I dream a lot. (T) (F)

215. I gasp for air when I sleep. (T) (F)

216. I have frequent nightmares. (T) (F)

217. I suffer from daily pain. (T) (F)

218. I use many over-the-counter painkillers. (T) (F)

219. I like to consult with my doctor about what medications to take. (T) (F)

220. I drink alcoholic beverages to numb my pain. (T) (F)

221. People care the way I feel. (T) (F)

222. Prescribed drugs always help more than they cause harm. (T) (F)

223. I use my own judgment as to how much medication to take. (T) (F)

224. Name all drugs and dosages you are taking.

____________________ ____________________
____________________ ____________________
____________________ ____________________
____________________ ____________________
____________________ ____________________
____________________ ____________________

225. What do doctors think is wrong with you?

____
____

226. What do you think is wrong with you?

____
____
____

227. Check all items that relate to you.

Anorexia_Arthritis_Asthma_Blooddisorders_ _ Bulimia _ Cancer_ Constipation_COPD_ Depression_Diabetes_Diarrhea_ Dizziness and fainting spells_Edema_ Chronic fatigue_ Fear of inherited diseases_Gastritis_ Hearing loss_Heart condition_ HIV_Hypertension_ _Injuries_Kidney disease_Liver disease_ Migraine_headaches_ Obesity_ Pregnancy_ Skin disease_ Sleep apnea _Chronic Urinary tract infections_ Vision disorders_ Difficulty walking_Others

MENTAL HEALTH

259.__________	264.__________
260.__________	274.__________
261.__________	262.__________
263.__________	275.__________
261.__________	266.__________
271.__________	276.__________
262.__________	267.__________
272.__________	277.__________
263.__________	268.__________
273.__________	278.__________

$$\frac{\text{32 QUESTIONS}}{\text{290 TOTAL QUESTIONS}} = 0.11 \text{ points}$$

$$\frac{\text{290 TOTAL QUESTIONS}}{160} = 1.81 = \text{MIPQ}$$

0.11X1.81=0.2079X100%=20.79 OR 21%

If 17 answers are True and
15 answers are False
The "ratio" would be 17/15
or 1.13x19.83=(22.41)%

228. I get gloomy for no reason. (T) (F)

229. I feel lonely even when there are people with me. (T) (F)

230. I daydream a lot and cry. (T) (F)

231. Life is too complicated, and I wish to die. (T) (F)

232. I get depressed for no reason. (T) (F)

233. I don't feel like doing anything. (T) (F)

234. It feels good to wake up every morning. (T) (F)

235. I truly deserve to live. (T) (F)

236. It is my fault that my family is suffering. (T) (F)

237. I hate to go to work. (T) (F)

238. School is not important in my life. (T) (F)

239. I am a valuable person to me and to society. (T) (F)

240. I hate when people tell me what to do. (T) (F)

241. I hate children. (T) (F)

242. When I get angry, I feel like punching someone. (T) (F)

243. When I am angry, I throw dishes, kick, hit, scream, and curse. (T) (F)

244. When another car passes me by on the road, I honk and curse him out. (T) (F)

245. Officials have no right to tell me how to live my life. (T) (F)

246. When someone walks on my lawn, I smile and say good day. (T) (F)

247. I am the only person to blame for my anger. (T) (F)

$$\frac{32 \text{ QUESTIONS}}{290 \text{ TOTAL QUESTIONS}} = 0.11 \text{ points}$$

$$\frac{290 \text{ TOTAL QUESTIONS}}{160} = 1.81 = \text{MIPQ}$$

0.11X1.81=0.2079X100%=20.79 OR 21%

If <u>17</u> answers are True and
15 answers are False
The "ratio" would be 17/15
or 1.13x19.83=(22.41)%

SPIRITUALITY

279.__________	285.__________
291.__________	297.__________
280.__________	286.__________
292.__________	298.__________
281.__________	287.__________
293.__________	299.__________
282.__________	288.__________
294.__________	300.__________
283.__________	289.__________
295.__________	301.__________
296.__________	302.__________
284.__________	290.__________

248. Prayer makes me feel better. (T) (F)

249. I really want to feel good. (T) (F)

250. I truly believe that I can get better. (T) (F)

251. I don't believe in God. (T) (F)

252. I don't believe in miracles. (T) (F)

253. I am afraid to die. (T) (F)

254. I believe in heaven and hell. (T) (F)

255. I turn to God in times of despair. (T) (F)

256. I don't have a loved one with whom to share my anguish. (T) (F)

257. I never thank God enough when I feel better. (T) (F)

258. It takes a strong willpower to deal with pain. (T) (F)

259. I accept changes in my life without doubting God. (T) (F)

260. People get sick at all ages. (T) (F)

261. There are sicker people than I. (T) (F)

262. I don't care about other people's faith. (T) (F)

263. Faith in God is important to me. (T) (F)

264. My family doesn't care if I am dead or alive. (T) (F)

265. The future scares me. (T) (F)

266. Faith and religion are the same. (T) (F)

267. Life means the union of the body, spirit, and soul. (T) (F)

268. Death means the end (T) (F)

269. Death means the separation of the body, spirit, and soul. (T) (F)

SCORES FOR GEDDI APTITUDE TEST

TODAY'S DATE____/_____/______

Name:__________________________ D.O.B.________/_______/_______ S.S.#________-________-________
Address:____

____

Telephone: (______)______/_________Cell:(______)______/_________
E-mail____

SUBJECT	QUANTITY	MAXIMUM	TOTAL (T)		TOTAL (F)			SCORE RATIO
PSYCHOSOCIAL	32	290	16	(F)	16	(T)	=	16/16= 1.0
NUTRITION	32	290	28	(F)	4	(T)	=	28/ 4= 7.0
LEISURE AND REC	32	290	21	(F)	11	(T)	=	21/11= 1.9
HYGIENE	32	290	2	(F)	30	(T)	=	2/30= 0.06
PHYSICAL HEALTH	24	290	2	(F)	22	(T)	=	2/22= 0.09
MENTAL HEALTH	20	290	4	(F)	6	(T)	=	14/ 6= 2.33
SPIRITUALITY	20	290	6	(F)	14	(T)	=	6/14= 0.42

RATIO: FALSE ANSWERS 89 (F) / TRUE ANSWERS 103 (T) =0.86 OR 86%

MENTAL HEALTH CHART

These scores are based on a study conducted on a group of:

200 normal functioning professionals
50 high school students
50 children with learning disabilities
25 children and adults with emotional disabilities
25 children and adults with mental retardation

The standard "Normal" group scored:	1.0+7.0 +1.9+0. 06+0.09+2.33+0.42	=12.8
The standard "Average" group scored:	2.0+1.5+3+1.5+1.5+3+2	=14.5
The standard "Emotional anxious" group scored:	2.5+2.5+4+2.5+3+4.5+3.5	=22.5
The standard "Mental disabled" group scored:	6+5+6+4.5+5.5+6.0+5.5	=23.2

The scores above indicate the level of alertness, anxiety, concerns, interests, mental status, and comprehension. The higher the scores, the higher is the anxiety or the disability.

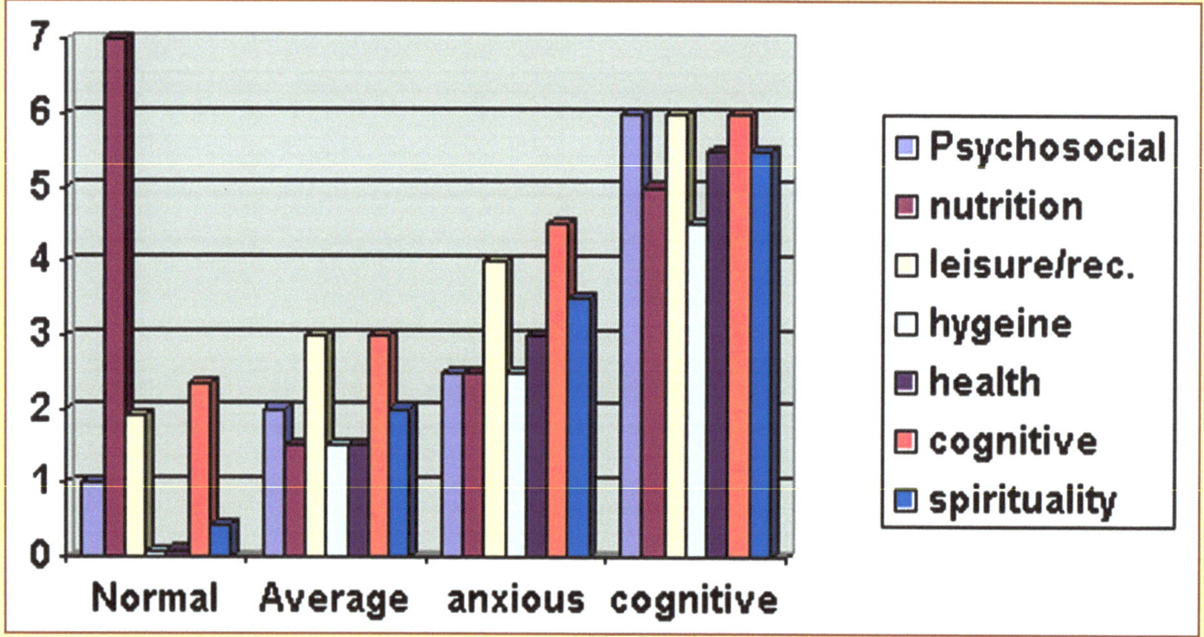

In the diagram above, we see a high anxiety level of 7 at the "normal" group for nutrition. This anxiety could be normal and healthy if the client wants to stay fit and well. Concerns, however, turn out to be when the client develops eating disorders, and becomes obsessed with his or her diets, and it affects his emotional and social life. People that could afford financially to pay for health clubs and for meals usually show this high anxiety level. A college student who wants to maintain high grades will show a higher level of anxiety than a C student. The normal group shows a normal rhythm with high-laws; and the final results show an average of 12.8, the lowest grade from the rest in the chart.

The mentally challenged show the highest score of 23.2. This indicates lack of concerns, lack of comprehension, lack of interests, and lack of awareness.

ACADEMIC CHART

The following chart shows the client's basic achievement scores as percentile rank. For example, a score of 85% means he or she scored higher than 85% of people tested for the same exam. Greater than 70 indicates strong will and interest in certain subjects. Less than 30 indicates lack of interest or dislike for certain activities. In the GEDDI exam, low scores are just as important as high scores. This can tell us the areas in which clients/students are weak, not interested, and their level of comprehension. It can also tell us how to help a student or a client to reach the maximum academic and psychological point.

Scale	Percentile	Percentage 0----10---20---30....40---50...60---70-- 80—90...100
Comprehension	98	
Reading	80	
Writing	50	
Mathematics	40	
Motor skills	70	
Psychosocial	20	
Concentration	25	
Social studies	80	
Nutrition	46	
Table games	90	
Science	5	
Arts and crafts	100	
Sports	45	

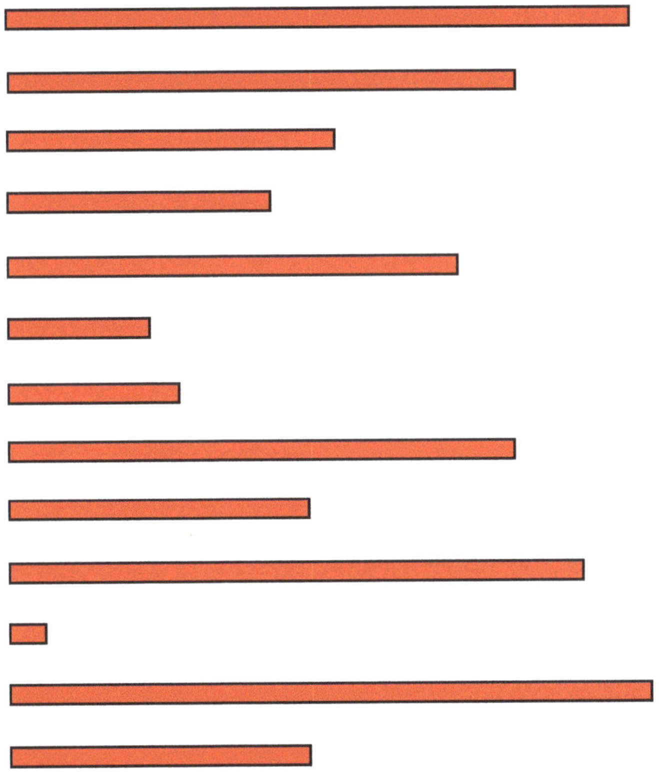

MOTOR SKILLS FOR THE CHALLENGED

Motor skills and child development are universally recognized, and it is every parent and teacher's responsibility to aid their children in motor skills development. It is easy and a great way to spend quality time with children. The way we measure motor skills is by age groups, disabilities, attention span, and by behavioral prototypes.

Fine motor skills are skills that allow a child to develop the ability to write and manipulate small objects.

Picking, brushing, painting, pulling, pushing, and lifting are all excellent tools to develop good motor skills. Toys must be appropriately sized for each child. We can also use finger painting, and painting with cotton or swabs. Coloring and scribbling allows children to develop their pincer grip needed for learning how to write.

With younger children, we can start them off with large peg puzzles. These puzzles have little knobs sticking out of each puzzle piece. This gives them more control over their finger movement. Another way to start off with children is by using larger blocks and moving slowly towards the smaller variety. The smaller the blocks, the more control they need to develop. Pushing small blocks too quickly will only get them frustrated, and they might give up.

Playing with Play-dough is another way to improve motor skills. Children roll it, cut it, and shape it. These activities are usually done in kindergarten, but it is also good for home activities.

Cutting papers helps to develop good motor skills because it requires a lot of coordination. Children can use plastic little scissors or even their fingers to cut papers or magazines.

Girls, more than boys, like to thread beads or pasta. This activity requires a lot of control and a steady hand.

Toddlers to adults use *gross motor skills* by running, jumping, hopping, etc. They require balance and coordination. Running is a game that requires moving quickly, and it encourages the development of gross motor coordination.

Climbing is a natural characteristic of children. Toddlers tend to climb chairs, tables, counters, and stairs. The more they climb, the better they are developing important gross motor muscles.

Gross motor skills are important for young and older people. Some of these motor skills include ball play, kicking, rolling, and throwing, which are some great ways to encourage gross motor development. A ball requires a little finer control. It has to be easily picked up and manipulated. Older kids might benefit from tennis, bowling, paddleball, batting, rocket ball, volleyball, soccer, and rope jumping. See below some examples of how to develop fine motor skills.

CHOOSE YOUR FAVORITE COLORS

1. Copy this design,

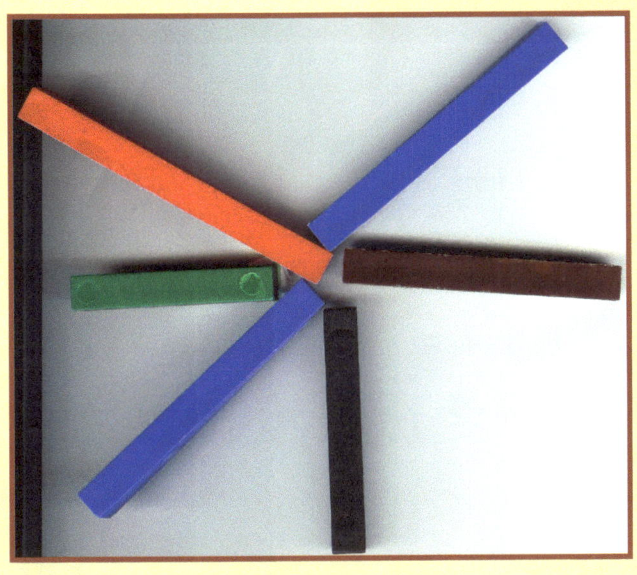

2. Memorize the shapes, and put them back in order.

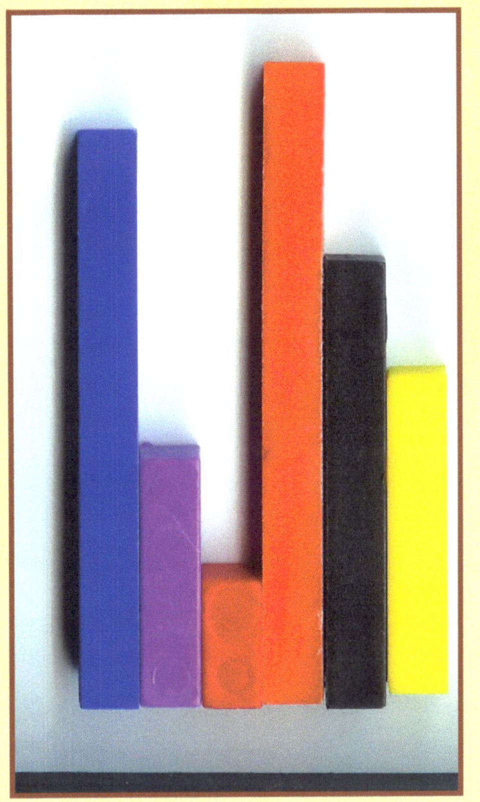

3. Copy this shape.

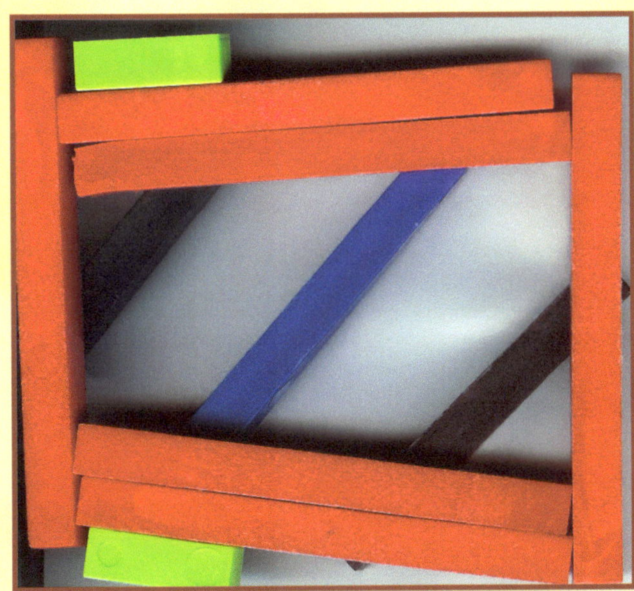

4. Build a house and a tree.

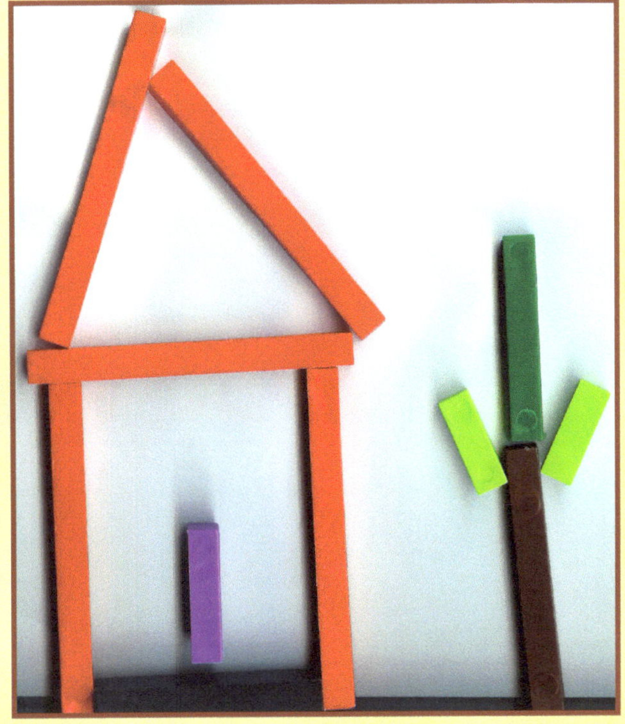

Use these pieces to copy the picture on the board.

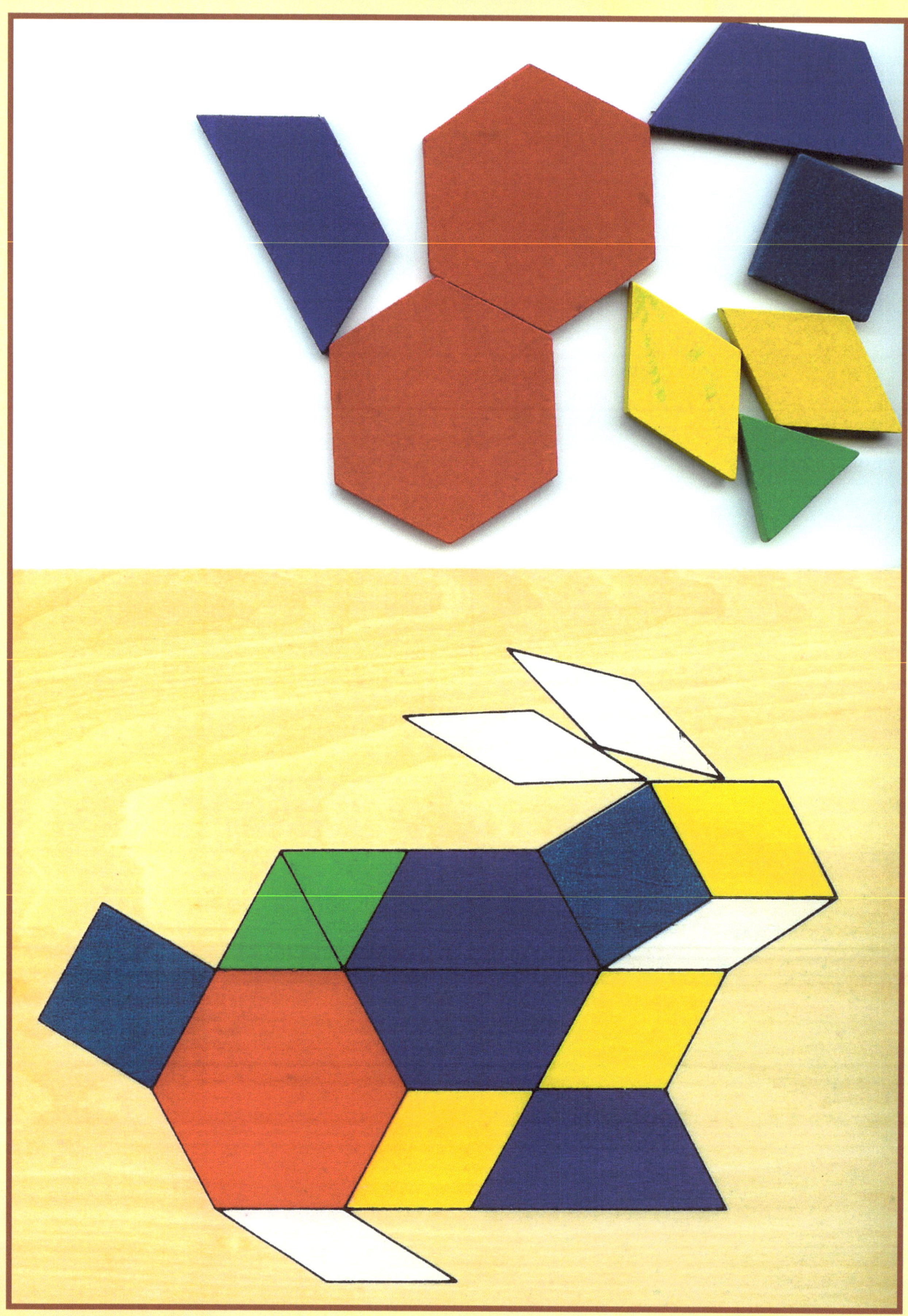

REVERSE IMAGE ANALYSIS (RIA)

picture I *Image 1* picture 2

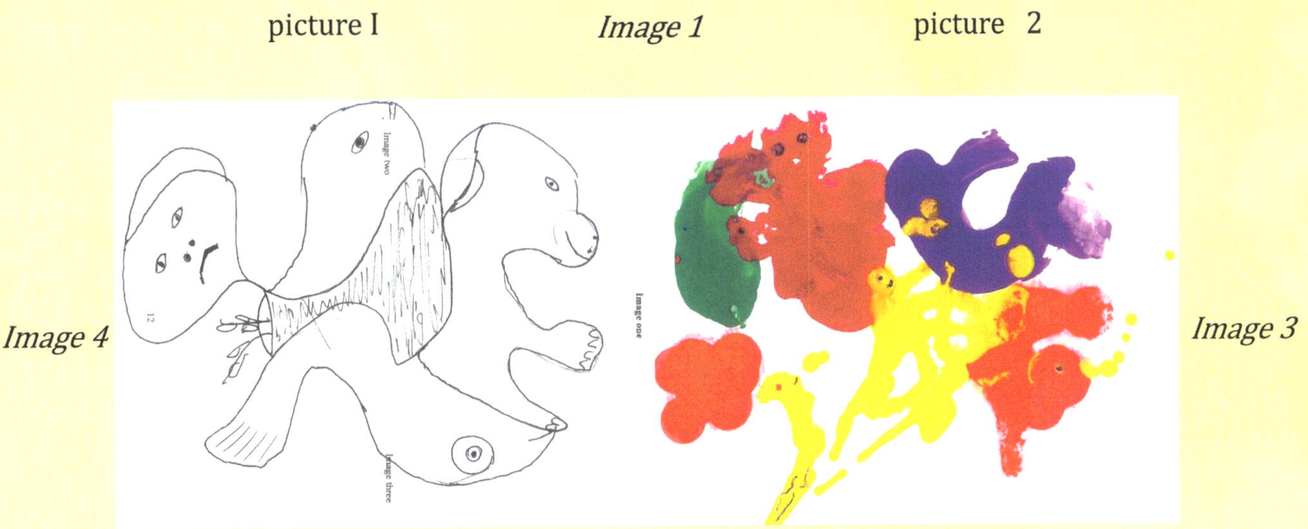

Image 4 *Image 3*

Image 2

The GEDDI **Reverse Image Analysis** (RIA) seeks to detect more than one reality to a given image in a form of art in order to apply it to the GEDDI study. Every person has at least two personalities: the good persona and the bad persona. The RIA helps the therapist detect hidden images behind a client's vision. People with Kookshrek Anxiety, Schizophrenia, Dyslexia, and those with phobias of different types, can bring forward the image they claim to see. In order to perform a picture of self-actualization, the client creates a non-specific energy drawing and painting.

In picture one, the therapist asked 17-year-old Jonathan to scribble. The therapist labeled: **Image I** on top, **Image II** on the bottom, **Image III** on the right, and **Image IV** on the left on a clean white paper as seen above. The client scribbled and then had to find images, enter eyes, and complete the figures that emerged in his vision. In Picture II, Jonathan spilled a thick layer of paint, and let it dry. When the paint dried, Jonathan inserted eyes, and identified at least two or more images in each angle. This showed the therapist the level of observance, creativity, imaginations, and if the client has specific phobias.

Both pictures demonstrate a worried individual who likes challenges, sports, and animals. However, he has a hard time reaching his goals. He feels insecure and always depends on others. Furthermore, he socially distances himself from society and prefers to spend leisure time outdoors, where he derives strength from nature. He feels most comfortable in the spring and on snowy days. The summer heat and the fall seasons are too threatening. During those months, Jonathan would stay at home most of the time. Jonathan shows early symptoms of Kookshrek Anxiety, and would have to take more tests to determine the severity of his disorder. More details are in the case studies section of this book.

SENSORY AWARENESS

We can often find children and adults to be behind in school because they lack the awareness of their own beings, surroundings, and their community. A 15-year-old girl was asked, "Besides food, what do you see in a supermarket?" She said, "I was never in a supermarket." Her mother replied, "Why do children have to go to a supermarket? I do all the shopping." This girl was in a second grade level instead of a high school level. The GEDDI focuses on sensory awareness and common sense more than regular education. Without these two areas, people cannot keep up with universal standards. Sensory awareness helps a person to get in touch with himself, and with reality.

Further, sensory awareness transcends a system of belief, discipline, and structure. It leads to immediate and direct experience through which we can discover and become a part of our natural ways of being and belonging.

We must first know ourselves before we can know others. How can we understand the feelings of others if we don't fully understand our own? By touching base with our everyday activities, we learn to accept others and ourselves. We must be self-oriented; be aware of our surroundings and understand the environment for individual growth and interpersonal relations; and be aware of societal and ecological issues in order to live a productive life.

The effort of self-awareness may begin simply by relaxing, tuning into our heartbeat, connecting with our breath, energies, and senses that bring us to a greater understanding of how we function in this world.

Through sensory awareness the client can learn how to tune in, reduce stress, derive energy conservation, structural economy, and more natural ways of being. It also teaches how one can see himself as a whole, and live to his maximum potentials.

Further, through sensory awareness, the client is able to become more aware of situations, think and perform more clearly, and live more fully in this world. It also helps the client to reclaim his/her natural being.

In the GEDDI model, Goldenthal uses a Sensory Awareness questionnaire to test the client's awareness. It is designed for therapeutic purposes and for self-discovery.

Goldenthal's theory on sensory awareness is based on the fact that the more the client is aware of situations, the more he opens up and is able to connect with himself, his immediate surroundings, and with the outside world that seems so estranged prior to this test. Below is a sample of a reality orientation test.

Scores for Sensory Awareness

1.________	16________	31________	46________	61________	76________
2.________	17________	32________	47________	62________	77________
3.________	18________	33________	48________	63________	78________
4.________	19________	34________	49________	64________	79________
5.________	20________	35________	50________	65________	80________
6.________	21________	36________	51________	66________	81________
7.________	22________	37________	52________	67________	82________
8.________	23________	38________	53________	68________	83________
9.________	24________	39________	54________	69________	84________
10.________	25________	40________	55________	70________	85________
11.________	26________	41________	56________	71________	86________
12.________	27________	42________	57________	72________	87________
13________	28________	43________	58________	73________	88________
14________	29________	44________	59________	74________	89________
15.________	30________	45________	60________	75________	90 ________

Total questions (90) ___ Total correct answers / Total answers = ____% 90/1 x _____/100% =___%

Example:

Total questions (90) 3 correct answers / 6 answers in each unit = 1/5 = 50% 90/1 x 50/100 = (45%)

Sum up all units

Divide total by 90 and get average score.

Add an equation in each unit.

Total questions (90) ___ ___ correct answers / answers in each unit = ____% 90/1 x _____/100% =___%

1. Besides shoes, what do you see in a shoe store?

1________________________
2________________________
3________________________
4________________________
5________________________
6________________________

2. Besides scissors and brushes, what do you see in a barbershop?

1________________________
2________________________
3________________________
4________________________
5________________________
6________________________

3. Besides food, what do you see in a supermarket?

1________________________
2________________________
3________________________
4________________________
5________________________
6________________________

4. Name three items you see in a hardware store.

1________________________
2________________________
3________________________

5. Besides drugs, what do you find in a pharmacy?
1____________________________
2____________________________
3____________________________
4____________________________
5____________________________
6____________________________

6. Give four reasons why school is important.
1____________________________
2____________________________
3____________________________
4____________________________

7. Besides bowling, what other activities do you do in a bowling alley?
1____________________________
2____________________________
3____________________________
4____________________________

8. Name four reasons why people go to a concert.
1____________________________
2____________________________
3____________________________
4____________________________

9. Besides cooking, what do you do in the kitchen?
1____________________________
2____________________________
3____________________________
4____________________________

10. What items do you store in a bathroom?
1____________________________
2____________________________
3____________________________
4____________________________
5____________________________
6____________________________

11. Name four activities you do in a park.
1____________________________
2____________________________
3____________________________
4____________________________

12. Besides water, name four things you see in the ocean.
1____________________________
2____________________________
3____________________________
4____________________________

13. What does jail mean to you?
1____________________________
2____________________________
3____________________________
4____________________________

14. Name four reasons why people go to a hospital.
1____________________________
2____________________________
3____________________________
4____________________________

15. What is a court?

____

16. Give four reasons why people go to a police station.
1____________________________
2____________________________
3____________________________
4____________________________

17. Name six good things you have at home.
1____________________________
2____________________________
3____________________________
4____________________________
5____________________________
6____________________________

18. Name six bad things you have at home.
1______________________________
2______________________________
3______________________________
4______________________________
5______________________________
6______________________________

19. Name six good things you see on the street.
1______________________________
2______________________________
3______________________________
4______________________________
5______________________________
6______________________________

20. Name six bad things you see on the street.
1______________________________
2______________________________
3______________________________
4______________________________
5______________________________
6______________________________

21. What does "table manners" mean to you?
1______________________________
2______________________________
3______________________________
4______________________________

22. Name people you must respect.
1______________________________
2______________________________
3______________________________
4______________________________
5______________________________
6______________________________

23. Besides bread, what items do you see in a bakery?
1______________________________
2______________________________
3______________________________
4______________________________
5______________________________
6______________________________

24. Name four things you fix.
1______________________________
2______________________________
3______________________________
4______________________________

25. Name four things you connect.
1______________________________
2______________________________
3______________________________
4______________________________

26. Name six forms of transportation.
1______________________________
2______________________________
3______________________________
4______________________________
5______________________________
6______________________________

27. Give six reasons why people celebrate.
1______________________________
2______________________________
3______________________________
4______________________________
5______________________________
6______________________________

28. Name four people you wish to write to, but you cannot because...
1______________________________
____
2______________________________
____
3______________________________
____
4______________________________
____

29. Name four people you would like to call and share your life with.
1______________________________
2______________________________
3______________________________
4______________________________

30. Name four people you really hate and wish they would be out of your life, and cite the reasons why.
1______________________________
____
2______________________________
____
3______________________________
____
4______________________________
____

31. Name four ancient forms of transportation
1____________________________
2____________________________
3____________________________
4____________________________

32. I wish I could help, but I cannot because...
____
____
____

33. I hate to______________________________
But I am forced to do it because
____
____

34. Give four reasons why you should change the way you dress.
1____________________________
2____________________________
3____________________________
4____________________________

35. I want to______________________________
But I cannot do it because...
____
____

THINGS I

36. Share with others:
1___________________________
2___________________________
3___________________________

37. Keep secrets from:
1____________________________
2____________________________
3____________________________
4____________________________
5____________________________
6____________________________
7____________________________

THINGS I TELL

38. My mom:
1____________________________
2____________________________
3____________________________

39. My dad:
1____________________________
2____________________________
3____________________________

40. A teacher:
1____________________________
2____________________________
3____________________________
4____________________________

41. A friend:
1____________________________
2____________________________
3____________________________
4____________________________
5____________________________

42. Doctor:
1____________________________
2____________________________
3____________________________
4____________________________

43. A nurse:
1____________________________
2____________________________
3____________________________
4____________________________

44. A lawyer:
1______________________
2______________________
3______________________
4______________________

45. A judge:
1______________________
2______________________
3______________________
4______________________
5______________________
6______________________

RULES YOU MUST FOLLOW AT

46. Home:
1______________________
2______________________
3______________________
4______________________

47. School:
1______________________
2______________________
3______________________
4______________________
5______________________

48. Court:
1______________________
2______________________
3______________________
4______________________
5______________________

49. Jail:
1______________________
2______________________
3______________________
4______________________
5______________________

50. Camp:
1______________________
2______________________
3______________________
4______________________

51. Hospital:
1______________________
2______________________
3______________________
4______________________

52. Train station
1______________________
2______________________
3 _____________________
4______________________
5______________________

53. On the street
1______________________
2______________________
3______________________
4______________________

54. Library
1______________________
2______________________
3______________________
4______________________

55. Department store
1______________________
2______________________
3______________________
4______________________

56. Restaurant.
1______________________
2______________________
3______________________
4______________________

57. Public restroom
1______________________
2______________________
3______________________
4______________________
5______________________

58. Things I want you to do when I

Cry ___________________________
Laugh _________________________
Scream ________________________
Isolate myself ___________________
Drink _________________________
Smoke _________________________
Hesitate_______________________
Run away______________________

59. Name ten crimes.

1_____________________
2_____________________
3_____________________
4_____________________
5_____________________
6_____________________
7_____________________
8_____________________
9_____________________
10____________________

60. Name six punishments

1_____________________
2_____________________
3_____________________
4_____________________
5_____________________
6_____________________

61. Name rewards you deserve and why?

1_____________________
____
2_____________________
____
3_____________________
____

62. Name an award you deserve and why.

____
____

63. Name 5 mistakes you did in the past, and you wish you had never done them. How would you correct the mistakes?

1_____________________
____
2_____________________
____
3_____________________
____
4_____________________
____
5_____________________
____

64. Name ten commitments to society

1_____________________
2_____________________
3_____________________
4_____________________
5_____________________
6_____________________
7_____________________
8_____________________
9_____________________
10____________________

65. Ten commitments to friends

1_____________________
2_____________________
3_____________________
4_____________________
5_____________________
6_____________________
7_____________________
8_____________________
9_____________________
10____________________

66. Ten commitments to relatives

1_____________________
2_____________________
3_____________________
4_____________________
5_____________________
6_____________________
7_____________________
8_____________________
9_____________________
10____________________

67. Ten commitments to G-d

1______________________________
2______________________________
3______________________________
4______________________________
5______________________________
6______________________________
7______________________________
8______________________________
9______________________________
10_____________________________

68. Ten commitments to yourself

1______________________________
2______________________________
3______________________________
4______________________________
5______________________________
6______________________________
7______________________________
8______________________________
9______________________________
10_____________________________

69. HOW TO PREPARE FOR A

Job interview

1______________________________
2______________________________
3______________________________
4______________________________
5______________________________
6______________________________

70. Court hearing

1______________________________
2______________________________
3______________________________
4______________________________
5______________________________

71. Administrator's position

1______________________________
2______________________________
3______________________________
4______________________________

72. Placement test

1______________________________
2______________________________
3______________________________
4______________________________

73. Staff meeting

1______________________________
2______________________________
3______________________________
4______________________________
5______________________________

74. Interviewing employees

1______________________________
2______________________________
3______________________________
4______________________________
5______________________________

75. Hiring volunteers

1______________________________
2______________________________
3______________________________
4______________________________
5______________________________

76. Get on time to work

1______________________________
2______________________________
3______________________________
4______________________________
5______________________________

77. Maintain positive attitude

1______________________________
2______________________________
3______________________________

Things you hear in the

78. Park

1____________________________
2____________________________
3____________________________
4____________________________
5____________________________

79. Airport

1____________________________
2____________________________
3____________________________
4____________________________
5____________________________

80. In the woods

1____________________________
2____________________________
3____________________________
4____________________________
5____________________________

81. Near the fireplace

1____________________________
2____________________________
3____________________________
4____________________________
5____________________________

82. In your room

1____________________________
2____________________________
3____________________________
4____________________________
5____________________________

83. In the gym

1____________________________
2____________________________
3____________________________
4____________________________
5____________________________

84. In the closet

1____________________________
2____________________________
3____________________________
4____________________________
5____________________________

85. In the backyard

1____________________________
2____________________________
3____________________________
4____________________________
5____________________________

86. In the ocean

1____________________________
2____________________________
3____________________________
4____________________________
5____________________________

87. In the sky

1____________________________
2____________________________
3____________________________
4____________________________
5____________________________

88. Things that move smoothly

1____________________________
2____________________________
3____________________________
4____________________________
5____________________________

89. Things that move down

1____________________________
2____________________________
3____________________________
4____________________________
5____________________________

90. Things that leak
1________________________
2________________________
3________________________
4________________________
5________________________

91. Things you pour
1________________________
2________________________
3________________________
4________________________
5________________________

92. Things that beat
1________________________
2________________________
3________________________
4________________________
5________________________

93. Things you hit

1________________________
2________________________
3________________________
4________________________
5________________________

94. The most important thing you wish to achieve in your life

____
____
____
____

95. Things you must do when you wake up in the morning

1________________________
2________________________
3________________________
4________________________
5________________________
6________________________
7________________________

96. Things you must do before you go to sleep
1________________________
2________________________
3________________________
4________________________
5________________________
6________________________
7________________________

SAFETY ACTIONS

97. When a friend falls, you call__________

98. When an animal is trapped in a hole, you call

____

99. Your friend is drunk and does not respond to you; you call ____________________

____

100. If your neighbor is overdosed with drugs, you call

____

101. What would you do if you witness a Robbery?

____

102. You are at a party with friends. The driver that drove you to the party is drunk, you don't have a driver's license, or your driver's license has been suspended. How would you get home?

1________________________
2________________________
3________________________
4________________________

103. Your parents lend you their car to go to a party, and your friend asks you to let her/him drive, what would you tell her/ him?
1.____________________________
2.____________________________
3.____________________________

104. Your friend lends you a car and you go into an accident, would you:
1. Just not tell her/him
2. Get to the nearest phone and call the police.
3. Take full responsibility to repair the car.
4. I will never accept the offer. I should never drive someone else's car unless it is a life-threateningsituation.

105. What would you do if you witness A crime?____________________________

106. What would you do if someone were smoking in bed____________________________

107. What would you do if someone is holding or playing with a gun?____________________________
____

108. What would you do if you see a child playing with pills?
1.____________________________
2.____________________________

109. What would you do if you see a child playing with matches? ____________________________
____

110. What would you do if you see someone choking?
1.____________________________
2.____________________________

111. What would you do if you suspect someone is having a heart attack?
1.____________________________
2.____________________________
3.____________________________

112. What would you do if you see smoke coming out of a house?
1.____________________________
2.____________________________
3.____________________________

113. What would you do if you suspect some one was cheating on you?

114. How should you react if, God forbid. you lose a loved one.
1.____________________________
2.____________________________
3.____________________________

115. What would you do if you see a child sitting on a window sill looking out?
1.____________________________
2.____________________________
3.____________________________

116. What do you do when you see your parents argue?
1.____________________________
2.____________________________
4.____________________________

117. What does love mean to you?
1.____________________________
2.____________________________
3.____________________________
4.____________________________

118. Name two people you really care for, and why?
1.____________________________
____
2.____________________________
____

SELF-AWARENESS

PERSONAL

119. Good looking Y N

120. Too tall for my age Y N

121. Too short for my age Y N

122. Just right for my age Y N

123. Too fat Y N

124. I love my hair Y N

125. I love my hair color Y N

126. I love my skin color Y N

127. I am healthy Y N

128. I am feeling good Y N

I LIKE TO

129. Learn from others Y N

130. Teach others Y N

131. Join clubs Y N

132. Join groups Y N

133. Act/model Y N

134. Volunteer Y N

135.Fly to space Y N

136. Become a millionaire Y N

137. Go to school Y N

138. Hang out with friends Y N

139. Associate with at least five friends Y N

140. Read Y N

141. Write Y N

142. Play outside Y N

143. Play a musical instrument Y N

144. Watch TV Y N

145. Dine out Y N

146. Hike in the woods Y N

147 Go to the circus Y N

148 Listen to music Y N

149 Eat with my family Y N

PEOPLE THAT CARE ABOUT ME.

150. Learn something new Y N

151. Paint Y N

152. Swim Y N

153. Play ball Y N

154. Shop Y N

155. Share Y N

156. Play with stuffed animals Y N

157. I like to help Y N

158. Travel to other countries Y N

159. My sister /s Y N

160. My brother/s Y N

161. my mother Y N

162 My father Y N

163. My teacher/s Y N

164. Grandparents Y N

165. Uncles/aunts Y N

166. My neighbors Y N

PSYCHOSOCIAL

I AM

167. Noisy Y N

168. Always happy Y N

169. Angry Y N

170. Hyperactive Y N

171. Talkative Y N

172. Disruptive Y N

173. Restless Y N

174. Lazy Y N

175. Nervous Y N

176. Anxious Y N

177. Short attention span Y N

THINGS I DO BUT SHOULD NOT

178. Fight Y N

179. Argue Y N

180. Scream Y N

181. Steal/shoplift Y N

182. Have sex Y N

183. Cheat Y N

184. Lie Y N

185. Take advantage Y N

186. Criticize Y N

187. Shadows Y N

188. Heights Y N

THINGS I AM AFRAID OF

189. Animals Y N

190. Trees/bushes Y N

191. Clouds Y N

192. When people stare at me Y N

193. Elevators Y N

194. Driving Y N

195. Travel/fly Y N

196. Wood cracking Y N

197. Germs Y N

198. Certain foods Y N

199. Water Y N

200. Night time Y N

201. Leave the house Y N

202. Large crowds Y N

203. Parents Y N

204. Rain Y N

205. Thunders Y N

206. Lightning Y N
207. Blood Y N
208. Demons Y N
209. Death Y N
210. War Y N
211. To stay home alone Y N
212. To go out in public Y N
213. To meet new people Y N
214. To take an exam Y N
215. To visit the dentist Y N
216. To visit a doctor Y N
217. To speak in public Y N
218. To eat in front of people Y N
219. To look good Y N
220. To sleep Y N
221. News reports Y N
222. G-d Y N
223. To sin Y N
224. End of the world Y N
225. Childbirth Y N
226. To marry Y N
227. To tell the truth Y N
228. Dreams and visions Y N
229. Disease Y N
230. Spouse Y N
231. Sibling Y N
232. Neighbor Y N
233. Teacher Y N
234. Others________________ Y N

THINGS I WANT

235. A car Y N
236. To make decisions Y N
237. Independence Y N
238. A mother in my life Y N
239. A father in my life Y N
240. To own a home Y N
241. To own a farm Y N
242. To own animals Y N
243. To own jewelry Y N
244. To own a car Y N
245. To fly a plane Y N
246. To become famous Y N
247. To be a rescue hero Y N

HEALTH AND HYGIENE

248. Shower daily Y N
249. Brush my teeth 2x a day Y N
250. Brush my hair daily Y N
251. Change clothes daily Y N

252. Change into pajamas Y N

253. Go to the dentist Y N

254. Go to the doctor Y N

255. Sleep enough hours Y N

256. Exercise Y N

257. Follow a healthy diet Y N

258. Relax on vacations Y N

259. School Y N

260. College Y N

261. Listen Y N

262. Communicate Y N

GOALS

263. Graduate from college Y N

264. Be an honest business person Y N

265. Be a professional Y N

266. Be a good parent Y N

267. Live comfortably financially Y N

268. Become an expert in a specific subject Y N

269. Become a leader Y N

SCORES: (Y) TRUE (N) FALSE

1__30__59____88__117__146__

2__31__60____89__118__147__

3__32__61____90__119__148__

4__33__62____91__120__149__

5__34__63____92__121__150__

6__35__64____93__122__151__

7__36__65____94__123__152__

8__37__66____95__124__153__

9__38__67____96__125__154__

10__39__68____97__126__155__

11__40__69____98__127__156__

12__41__70____99__128__157__

13__42__71__100__129__158__

14__43__72__101__130__159__

15__44__73__102__131__160__

16__45__74__103__132__161__

17__46__75__104__133__162__

18__47__76__105__134__163__

19__48__77__106__135__164__

20__49__78__107__136__165__

21__50__79__108__137__166__

22__51__80__109__138__167__

23__52__81__110__139__168__

24__53__82__111__140__169__

25__54__83__112__141__170__

26__55__84__113__142__171__

27__56__85__114__143__172__

28__57__86__115__144__173__

29__58__87__116__145__174__

175__204__233__262__

176__205__234__263__

177__206__235__264__

178__207__236__265__

179__208__237__266__

180__209__238__267__

181__210__239__268__

182__211__240__269__

183__222__241__

184__213__242__

185__214__243__

186__215__244__

187__216__245__

188__217__246__

189__218__247__

190__219__248__

191__220__249__

192__221__250__

193__222__251__

194__223__252__

195__224__253__

196__225__254__

197__226__255__

198__227__256__

199__228__257__

200__229__258__

201__230__259__

202__231__260__

203__232__261__

THINGS THAT ANNOY

_ Birds
_ Clenching teeth
_ Controlling people
_ Ducks
_ Mosquitoes
_ Fidgeting
_ Flies
_ Grouchy people
_ Slurping
_ Whining
_ Someone talking over your shoulder
_ Someone reading next to you
_ Snoring
_ Someone staring at you
_ Someone talking when you are talking
_ Liars
_When people are too honest
_When someone gives you orders
_When people take advantage of you
_ People that borrow things all the time
_ People that visit too often
_ Grinding teeth
_ When someone swallows loudly
_The touch of sand
_A dripping faucet
_The noise of footsteps
_When someone knows better than you
_The noise of crunching papers or leaves
_Sound of an airplane
_Sound of a car horn
_When people give you advice
_When someone tells you the truth
_To obey rules
_Someone playing with his or her hair
_When people are calling daily to check on you
_Junk mail
_Traveling
_Reading a book
_Sitting in school
_Getting up in the morning
_An alarm clock
_Planning a daily schedule
_Cleaning your room
_Helping at home
_When the phone rings
_Waiting on line
_Listening to a lecture
_Someone picking his or her teeth
_Taking daily showers
_When people are too noisy in the morning
_Paying bills
_Sitting in a doctor's waiting room
_Stupid people
_Someone chewing gum
_People that are always neat
_Cleaning daily
_Parents
_Children
_Siblings
_Bosses/controllers
_Small salaries
_Paying taxes
_Bank tellers
_Honking cars
_Con artists
_Two-faced people
_Frequent apologies
_Frequent thank you's
_Nosy people
_Gossiping
_Co-workers
_Flies/mosquitoes/bees
_Music
_Rain/snow/winds
_Public transportation
_Boredom
_Life
_Frequent illnesses
_Staying home for too long
_Watching someone biting nails
_Dressing formally
_Parties
_People walking barefoot
_Itching
_Dandruff
_People spitting on the street
_Taking walks
_Running errands
_Smoking in public
_Prostitutes in your neighborhood
_Promises that are never delivered
_Politicians
_News reports
_Slandering

LIST TEN SCENTS YOU LIKE

1_____________________________________
2_____________________________________
3_____________________________________
4_____________________________________
5_____________________________________
6_____________________________________
7_____________________________________
8_____________________________________
9_____________________________________
10_____________________________________

LIST TEN ODORS YOU HATE

1_____________________________________
2_____________________________________
3_____________________________________
4_____________________________________
5_____________________________________
6_____________________________________
7_____________________________________
8_____________________________________
9_____________________________________
10_____________________________________

LIST TEN FLAVORS YOU LIKE

1_____________________________________
2_____________________________________
3_____________________________________
4_____________________________________
5_____________________________________
6_____________________________________
7_____________________________________
8_____________________________________
9_____________________________________
10_____________________________________

LIST TEN FLAVORS YOU HATE

1_____________________________________
2_____________________________________
3_____________________________________
4_____________________________________
5_____________________________________
6_____________________________________
7_____________________________________
8_____________________________________
9_____________________________________
10_____________________________________

LIST TEN THINGS YOU LIKE TO TOUCH

1_____________________________________
2_____________________________________
3_____________________________________
4_____________________________________
5_____________________________________
6_____________________________________
7_____________________________________
8_____________________________________
9_____________________________________
10_____________________________________

LIST TEN THINGS YOU HATE TO TOUCH

1_____________________________________
2_____________________________________
3_____________________________________
4_____________________________________
5_____________________________________
6_____________________________________
7_____________________________________
8_____________________________________
9_____________________________________
10_____________________________________

NEUROLOGICAL COMMANDS

1. Look at my eyes.
2. Touch my nose, and then touch the tip of your nose.
3. Look up.
4. Look down.
5. Look to your right.
6. How many fingers do you see?_______
7. Now_________
8. And now_____
9. Blink your eyes five times.
10. Lift your eyebrows.
11. Turn your head to the right.
12. Turn your head to the left.
13. Bend your head down to your chest.
14. Tilt your head back.
15. Bend down, and touch your left toe.
16. Stretch your arms to the front.
17. Lift your left hand above your head.
18. Put your left arm behind your left neck.
19. Stretch your right arm backward.
20. Put your left arm down.
21. Touch your right shoulder with your left hand.
22. Swing your left arm.
23. Swing your right arm.
24. Swing both arms together
25. Kick your right foot.
26. Kick your right foot backward.
27. Kick your left foot forward.
28. Touch your left shoulder with your right hand.
29. Count back from 38 to 20.
30. Count back by two's from 40-24.
31. Count back in three's from 27-0.
32. Jump up three times.
33. Jump down five times.
34. How do you push a heavy box?
35. How do you pull a wagon?
36. How do you pick apples?
37. How do you pick spinach?
38. If you jump forward three steps
    jump back five steps
    jump to the right eight steps
    jump to the left three steps
    jump forward nine steps
39. How many steps did you jump altogether?

    ____
40. How many times did you jump up and down?__________________________
41. How many times did you jump to the right and to the left?

COMMENTS

SELF EXPRESSION AND HANDWRITING ANALYSIS

Write a one-page essay about a dream that you remember well. If you don't remember any dream, make up a dream. Use the back to complete the essay if you need more space.

NAME:____________________________________

GENDER: MALE FEMALE

DATE OF BIRTH:______/_______/_________

HAND USED TO WRITE THIS ESSAY: (RIGHT) (LEFT) (BOTH)

CREATIVE WRITING

LIST 20 WORDS THAT POP INTO YOUR MIND

USE THESE WORDS IN ORDER TO WRITE AN ESSAY. UNDERLINE THE WORDS FROM THE LIST.

1_______________________
2_______________________
3_______________________
4_______________________
5_______________________
6_______________________
7_______________________
8_______________________
9_______________________
10_______________________
11_______________________
12_______________________
13_______________________
14_______________________
15_______________________
16_______________________
17_______________________
18_______________________
19_______________________
20_______________________

GOLDENTHAL EYE DRAWING DIAGNOSTIC IMAGING

The Goldenthal Eye Drawing Diagnostic Imaging is designed to help counselors analyze individuals' causes of fear, and to help the client come face to face with images that trigger visions and phobias. Just like any other psyche evaluation, the *GEDDI* uses drawings, scribbles, photography, and paintings to diagnose and cure patients with the *Kookshrek* Anxiety Disorder; and to diagnose those with psychosis, other delusions, and phobias. The therapist uses both ancient healing methods to remove the spell of the *evil eyes*, and spiritual endeavors caused by this disorder. Scores cannot measure the Geddi. The way we score it is by the reaction of the client during episodes, progress of mental and physical status, and by psychosocial changes. The following examples were taken from one hundred men, women, and children. They were chosen randomly or during therapeutic sessions. Studies show that Kookshrek Anxiety begins at birth, and men and women equally suffer from it. However, women are more likely to become healers and seem to be able to control the disorder. They learn early in life to remove the spell of the evil eye. Men have a harder time coping with the situation. They express their fears with anger and would most likely refuse to seek help. Let us see some samples of these tests.

TELEPHONE ANALYSIS

The telephone analysis is designed to analyze a patient's memory, level of anxiety, personalities, characteristics, energy level, intuitions, and artistic skills. For example: Use a telephone number that you know by heart and that you use frequently. Connect the numbers without lifting your pencil. Put a dot next to the numbers. Should a number appear more than once, trace a small line and place a dot next to that number.

Telephone: (   ) ________-__________

DIAGRAM ONE			DIAGRAM TWO			DIAGRAM THREE		
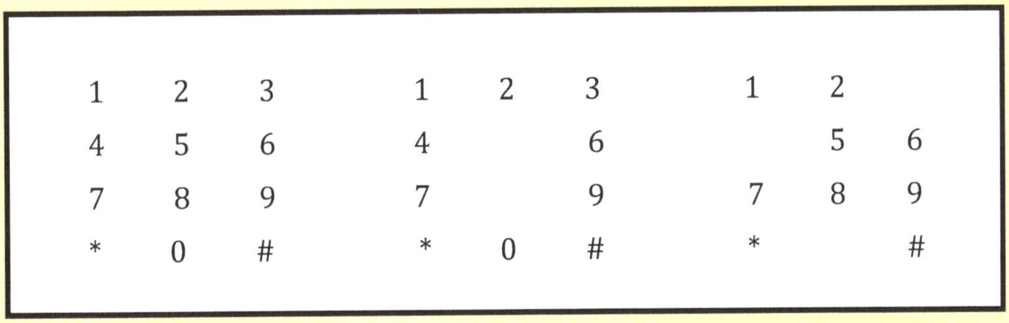 1	2	3	1	2	3	1	2	
4	5	6	4		6		5	6
7	8	9	7		9	7	8	9
*	0	#	*	0	#	*		#

DIAGRAM FOUR			DIAGRAM FIVE			DIAGRAM SIX
	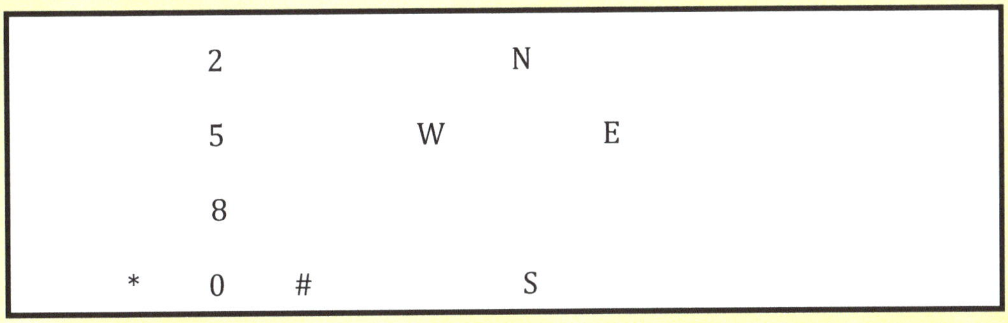 2			N		
	5		W		E	
	8					
*	0	#		S		

Fill in the numbers and symbols as it appears on your telephone.

Fill in the letters as it appears on your telephone.

Fill in the numbers and letters as it appears on your telephone.

COMMENTS:

SELF IMAGE MODEL

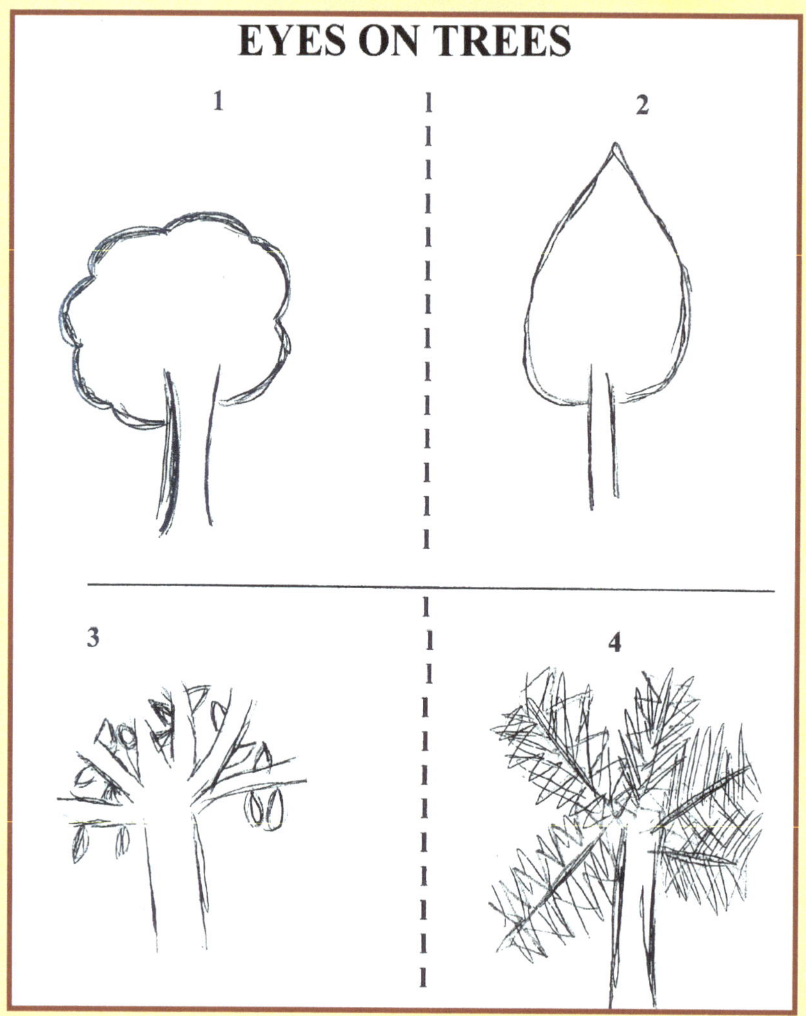

These pictures fit into the Self Image Model category. In this case a fifteen-year-old female feels no self-value nor is she aware of her appearance or her environment. These pictures give the counselor an idea of how the client values herself, and how much she is aware of her environment, her imagination, creativity, self-image, and self awareness. The client was instructed to draw one type of tree as follows:

Picture one: draw a trunk of a tree only.

Picture two: insert leaves.

Picture three: draw fruits.

Picture four: finalize the picture. Feel free to draw grass around the tree, a bird, or anything to enhance the tree.

Picture one: The counselor ordered the client to draw one type of a tree in all four pictures beginning with the trunk only. She inserted the first trunk of the tree in picture number one, but immediately finalized the drawing without developing branches, leaves, fruits, or the surroundings around the tree as she was instructed.

Picture two: The therapist reminded the client of the first instruction, but once again, the client completed the tree with a diagram that resembles a leaf.

Picture three: In picture three, the counselor reminded the client to stick to the original instruction. This time, the client inserted thick branches, short in size, with minimal curving. There are no leaves on either branch, but there are fruits. Even though there are fruits on the tree, there is no sign of life. Once again, picture three is not consistent with the first two pictures. So far, all three pictures represent different characteristics.

Picture four: shows a different picture all together. This tree has branches and leaves. The twigs appear like stiff sticks. The leaves are rough, but they complete the tree. There is no grass, birds, or any additional characteristics to enhance the tree.

Conclusions

The pictures above show a person with poor imagination. She is a loner, a hard learner, has no common sense, poor reality orientation, is not aware of her environment, and one that must be constantly encouraged and motivated. She has difficulties following commands, and her self-image is extremely poor.

At this time, this client is comfortable with the minimal information she obtains about her surroundings and education. She does not seek more information, and education is not an important factor in her life. The client has no goals and lives day by day with what she has.

This client has a short attention span and likes to complete projects immediately. She can concentrate on one thing at a time. Quantity is more important to her than the quality of a project. She derives immediate gratification from a complete project and does not worry for later. The tree clearly represents this girl's image. Just like the short stems on the tree, the girl is short, obese, and her limbs are shorter than usual.

SCRIBBLE ANALYSIS TEST

The GEDDI **Scribble Analysis Test** is the tunnel that leads to one's soul. It is easy, quick, and it represents a person's inner and outer lifestyle from his inner struggles to resolution. It also tells a person's history from the past to the present. In **Scribble Analysis**, the client sits comfortably near a table and scribbles on a clean white paper with a pencil. The therapist labels **Image 1** north of the paper; **Image 2**, south of the paper; **Image 3**, east of the paper; and **Image 4**, west of the paper. She then observes the client's movements, shapes, tightness, looseness, rhythm or flow, location, and direction of scribbles. When the client completes the test, the therapist analyzes the scribble in a clockwise direction and documents the findings from Images:

(1-3), (3-2), (2-4), (4-1). See figure.

CLOCKWISE READING

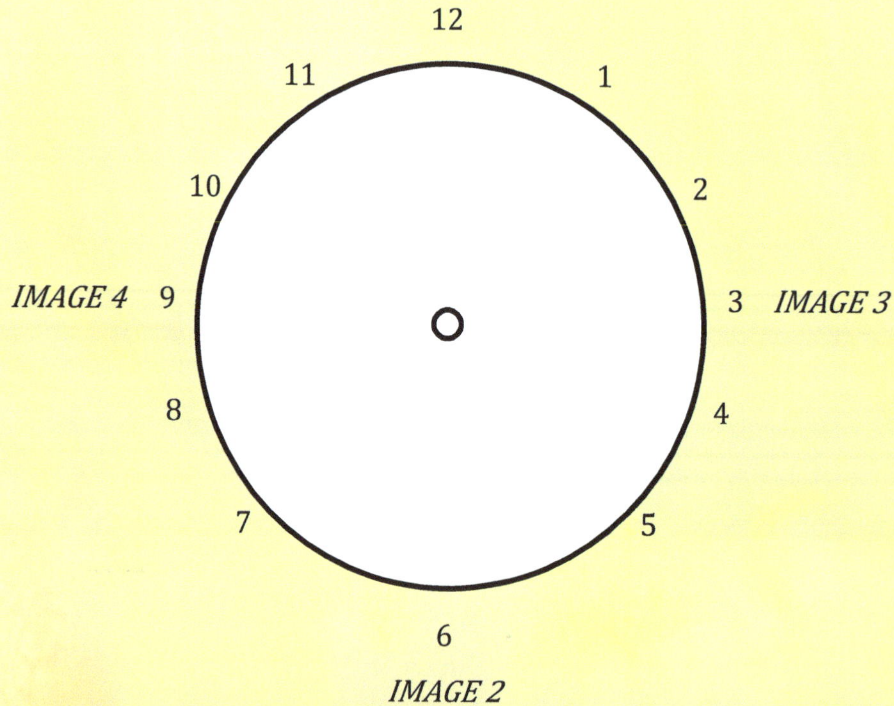

SAMPLE OF SCRIBBLE ANALYSIS

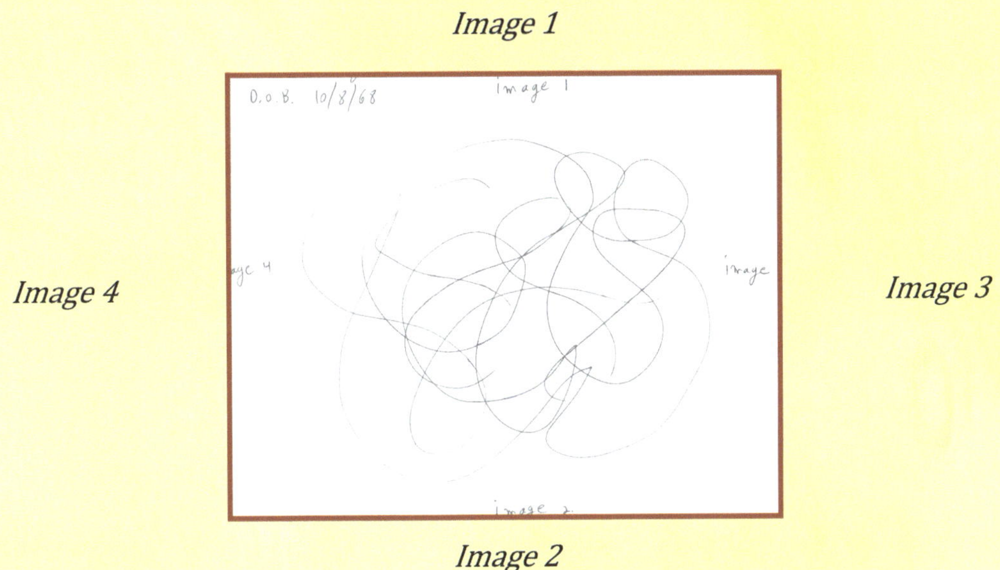

For a more accurate reading, a scribble analysis should be drawn with a pencil only on a white clean paper. This scribble demonstrates a friendly, pleasant individual that depends on others to make decisions for her. She does not like to take on responsibilities and would often blame others for her failure. She has a short temper; she likes to promise things, screams, and threatens, but is harmless. She never keeps her promises, and her threats are in vain. Such a person does not take care of house chores, does not make efforts to bring home money, and would often expect others to provide for her. She also tends to tell others about her issues and expects sympathy. This diagram shows that this individual has good intentions, but never pursues. She shows some rhythm of life, which apparently keeps her going. As you can see, there are too many ends on the scribble, which indicates that she has many unsolved issues. She gives up easily and gives in to whomever tries to take advantage of her. This is an illiterate woman who lives presently in the past. She makes no efforts to achieve goals and lives day by day on charity of others. In other words, she is a freeloader.

THE GEDDI ENERGY PAINTINGS

ATOMIC SAMPLE

An atomic sample is taken from a complete picture when the therapist suspects that the client withholds important information.

PICTURE ONE

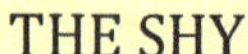

THE SHY

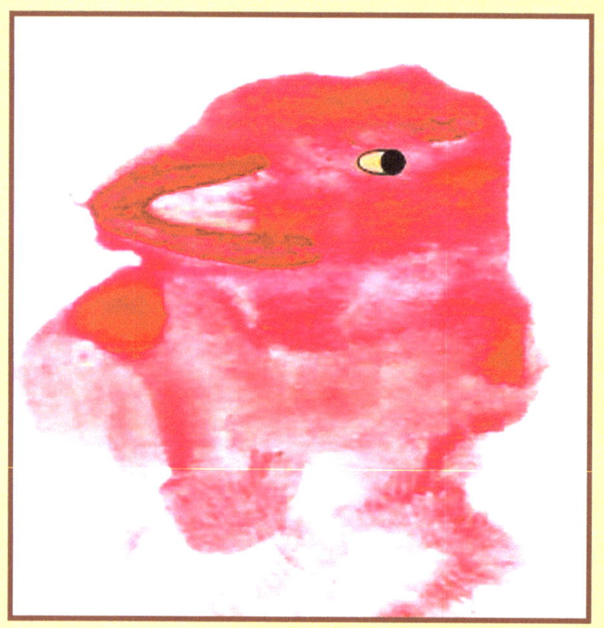

Picture one represents an individual with a low self- image and low value. He or she fails to value the good things he or she has accomplished in life. He feels unsettled and unfulfilled, even though he has accomplished more than others. His split lip and his toothless mouth show that he cannot speak up for his rights. When it comes to speak up for friends and family members, he would speak up with no fear. There is one big heavy tooth that goes back to the rear of the head. This demonstrates a strong individual who is committed to his family and all responsibilities. He or she is honest and modest.

The diagram shows a calm, happy educated person who likes to explore a variety of non-specific subjects, and is multi-talented. However, due to health issues, and financial tribulations, he or she cannot pursue plans and goals. As a result, this would often put him or her into episodes of depression and outbursts.

PICTURE TWO

The Hunter

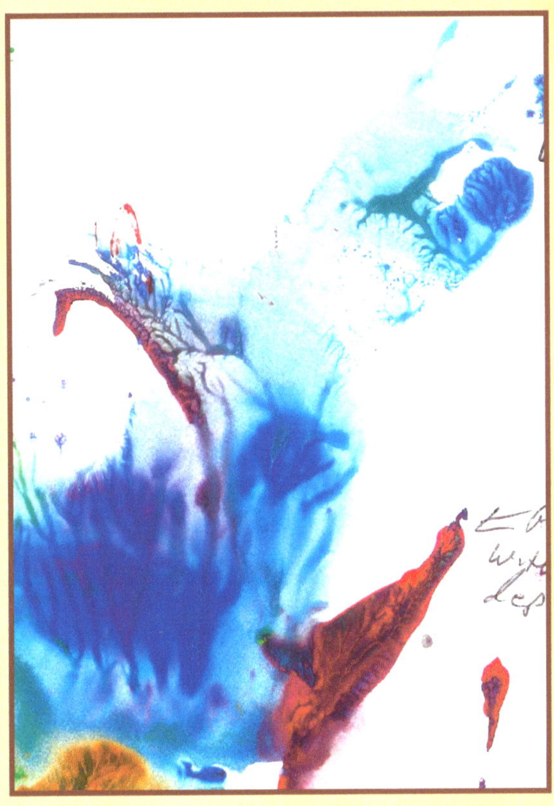

Picture two demonstrates an animal lover. He likes to experiment, but does not like to share his findings with others. This man is possessed with evil thoughts and gets angry easily. Also, this figure illustrates a talented comedian and an excellent actor. In real life, it is hard to get along with him. He is a loner and does not associate with friends. If you take a closer look, you can see snakes and venom sticking out in many angles. His insides are exposed, and you can see his ribs and arteries very clearly as if looking through a glass. This shows a person with multiple personality disorders. Although he appears strong and masculine, he is physically and mentally very sick. Also, such a person tends to be delusional and lives in constant fear. He hears and sees demons, and always feels as if someone is following him. Therefore, he is not responsible for his actions. He does not intend to hurt anyone, but it could happen if he thinks that a demon was there to attack him. This person does not get married nor does he live with a woman. He believes that being sexually active with a woman is like having sex with a demon. However, in his mind and in his dreams, he is sexually intimate with demons.

PICTURE THREE

HEALTH CRISIS

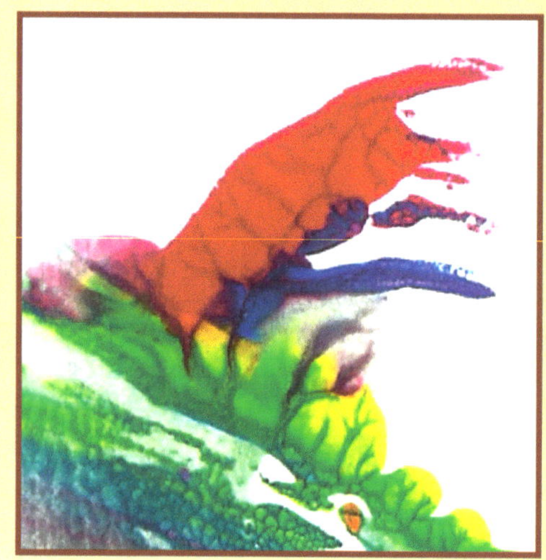

Picture number three is an atomic sample taken from a complete picture. The character in this picture shows clearly a dual personality. One is his strength and his wish to live. And the other shows a fragile, ill person. To the upper right, we can see a huge body with a snake-like looking penis. This body is positioned in the wrong place, but it is there for a reason. The heart is not visible. But the color of the heart, and the arteries and veins are clearly visible. It also indicates that this person speaks from his heart and tries to reach out to someone. Since there is no other significant around him, he uses his inner spirit to communicate. Therefore, his heart appears as a body with edges stretching out.

Further, this picture has similar characteristics as picture number two in which he feels possessed by demons that chew his life away. Even though he has strong sexual desires, he is most likely impotent and suffers from having stones in the urinary tract. His condition causes him a great deal of anxiety and rage. But he has no one to project his frustration to.

Below and in the back of the red body on the right, we see cloudy organs, most likely his lungs. The color and shape of the lungs show a smoker with early signs of lung cancer. Below the blue organ, we see cloudy and inflamed arteries, which suggests that this individual has moderate to severe renal stenosis.

To the left, we see a multitude of cells or plaque. His blood flow is thick, and the circulation is poor. This character tires easily, keeps isolated, and often feels on the downside. To the right, even though the overall condition is poor, there is hope. At the time of this exam, the left appears more life threatening.

This person is modest, but not too shy to reveal his problems. He seeks help and is willing to comply with medical caregivers.

We referred this client for medical attention, energy therapy, and for a psyche evaluation. Purification of his blood to remove all his toxins is highly recommended.

PICTURE FOUR

THE SHARPER IMAGE

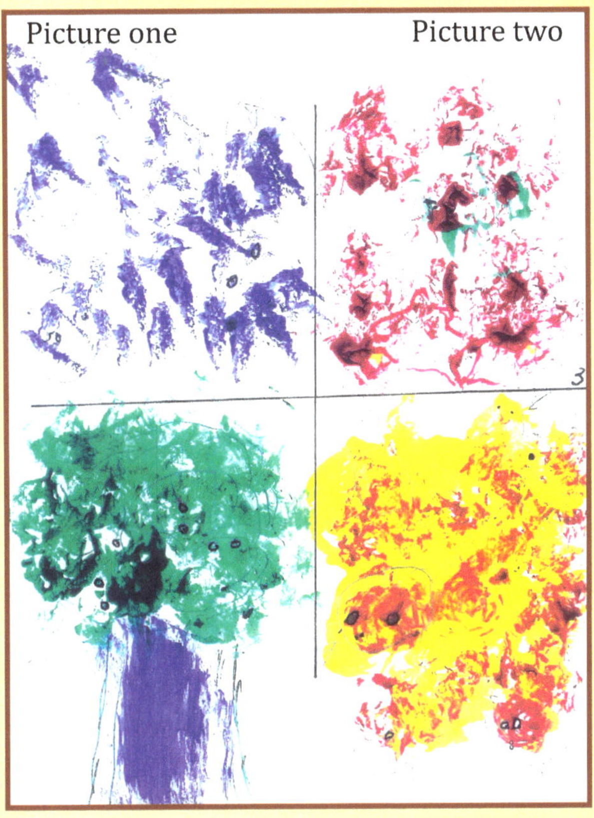

Picture three Picture four

All four portraits were painted with sponges and water paints. These pictures show a very disturbed individual. He is delusional, satanic, and worships witches. He does not show affection, and people are afraid to be in his area. This person does not see the real world. He sees only evil. He studies witchcraft and belongs to dangerous groups.

Picture one tells us that this client lives in a different world than the rest of us. He has little or no connection to our universe. He is a dreamer, delusional, and very fearful. No one can convince him that his hallucinations are not real.

Picture two shows an individual who is afraid of insects and pests. He sees them even when others near him tell him that there are no insects or mice around him. They appear everywhere. This person is filthy and poorly groomed. He seems to be heavily into drugs, and he is trapped in fear.

Picture three shows a possessed tree with evil eyes everywhere. This might present an individual with Kookshrek Anxiety, and the tree could be the cause of his bizarre behavior.

Picture four demonstrates a person who is afraid of fire. His nightmares are from his past life where several people in his family were probably burned. He is still reliving this tragedy and cannot separate his present life from his past. This frightened and confused individual must undergo extensive counseling and psychiatric care.

WASH PAINT

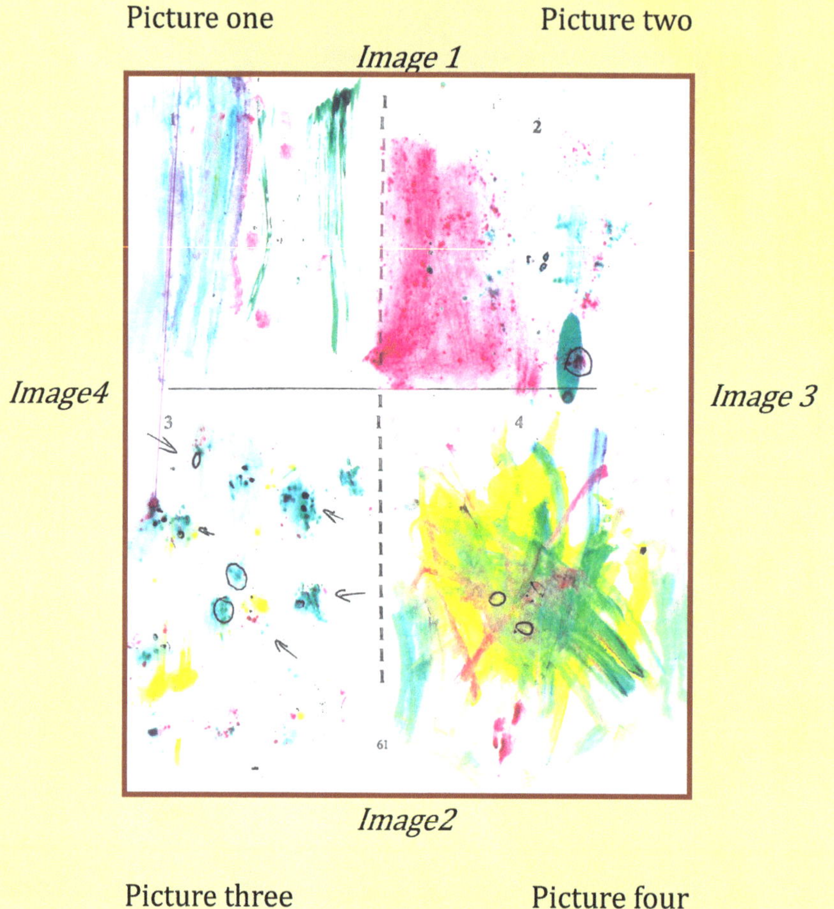

For these pictures the client uses a thin brush, water paint, and a pencil. The client can smear, create lines, splash, and finally insert eyes to create images.

The findings in these pictures demonstrate a lazy individual with poor artistic skills and a poor imagination. Based on these paintings, his or her learning capacity is poor, and he/she has a short attention span and poor concentration.

Further, this individual is a chronic liar and tends to bend the truth even when caught in a lie.

Picture three shows many eyes. This indicates paranoia. Picture four shows confusion and instability. The lines have no direction and are untidy. There are several meaningless images. The client sees the center of the picture as a face of a creature, but in reality he or she knows that this is an imaginary image. This can suggest an individual with emotional problems who lives with no rules.

PICTURE SIX

THE MADMAN

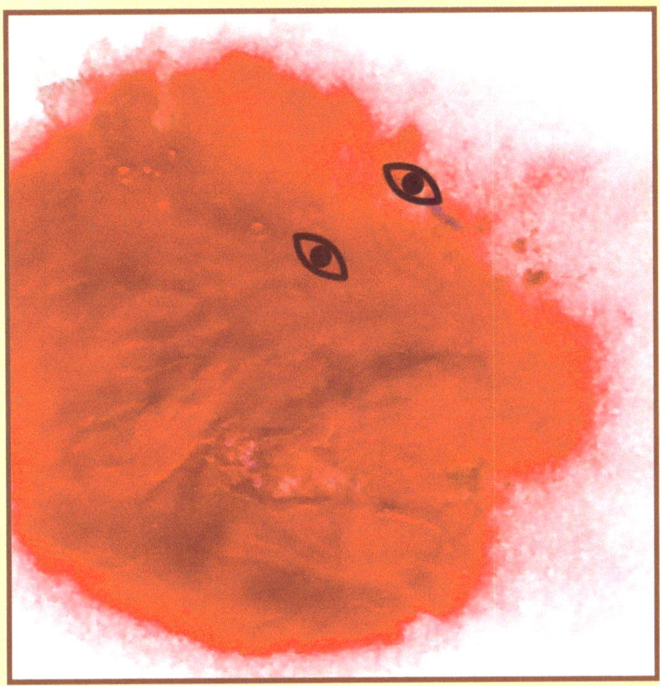

Picture six: This forty-eight-year-old male was going to use cotton balls and oil paint to create a picture. Some of the paint spilled, and the client got frustrated and refused to try again. However, he was willing to darken the eyes to create an image. This diagram was used as an **energy-painting** test to diagnose his mental status. His wife of two years can no longer tolerate his behavior and wants to bring some healing into their home.

This energy painting demonstrates a mad, angry individual that likes to control and manipulate the world. Such an individual believes that he is king of his household, king of his community, and king of the universe. No one tells him what is right or wrong.

Further, this individual hates to work and prefers to sit on a couch, nibble, and command others to do things for him. He hates to dress for special events and tends to be on the obese side.

Mr. Madman minds everyone's business, but cannot take care of his own. He does not settle with anyone for anything. He makes all the decisions. He has no sense of humor and always feels that he has to punish the world.

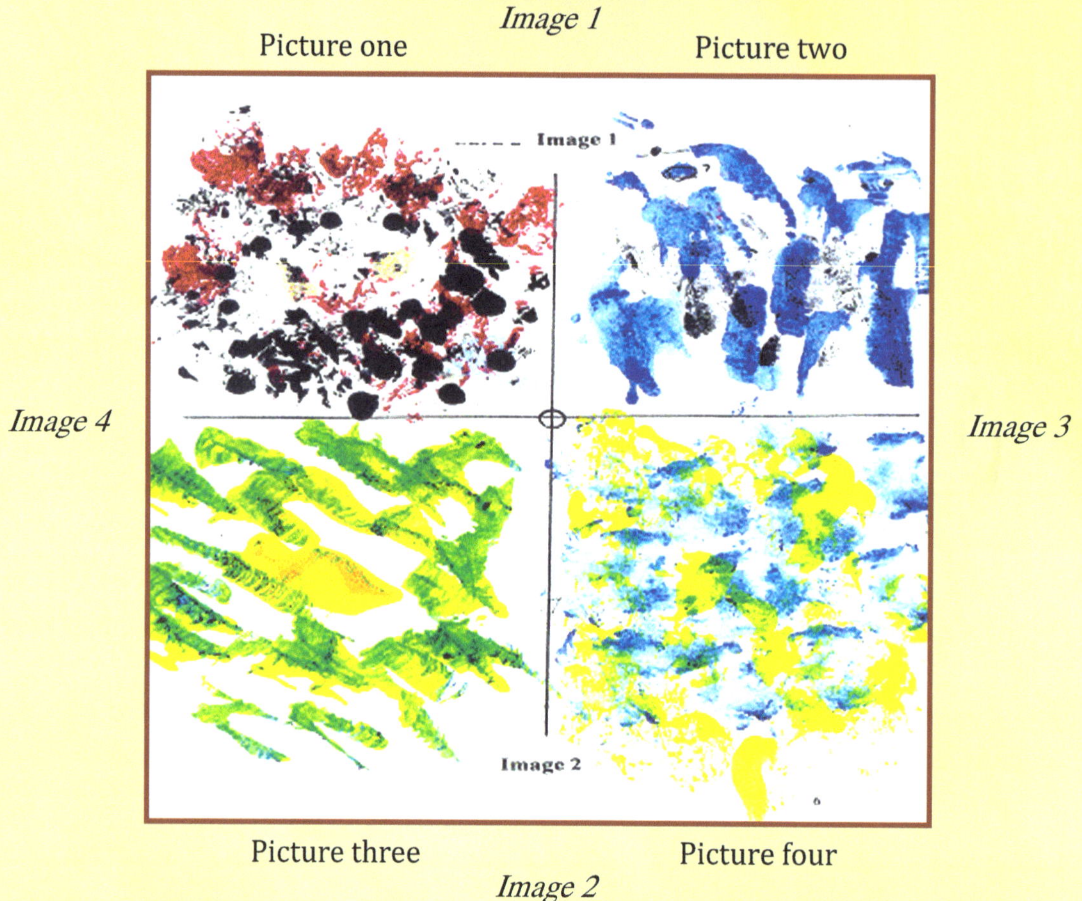

For these paintings, this female client used water paint and oil paint, colors of choice, a toothbrush, Q-tip, and cotton balls. She splashed, sprayed, doted, smeared, and stroked the paint.

The client sat comfortably next to the table. The counselor displayed the paints and tools she could use for these paintings. Further, the counselor labeled **Image 1** on top, **Image 2** on the bottom, **Image 3** on the right, and **Image 4** on the left. This helps the counselor read the final pictures from all angles. This test is used to diagnose causes of fears, confusion, and spiritual connections to specific beliefst.

Picture one demonstrates an insecure woman that must belong to a small, organized sect in order to belong, and for security reasons. These kinds of people are afraid of the unknown, the end of the world, fear war, fear starvation, and fear death. By belonging to a messianic group, they feel relief and a sense of redemption. They would do anything to get close to the "Messiah" who promises to bring salvation. David Koresh, in Waco, Texas, claimed to be the Messiah and protected his people by supplying them with ammunition, food, clothing, and everything they needed in case the world was coming to an end. Another group believed in a man named Applebaum who claimed to be the redeemer. In the early 90s when comet Hail-Bob appeared near planet Earth, he told them that the comet came to take them to a safer world. Thirty-eight followers, dressed in uniforms, committed suicide because they believed what their leader told them. Among them were hard working intelligent people. There is a Jewish cult named Lubavitch, or Chabbad. They bring together people from all faiths who were once confused, on drugs, were convicts, and homeless. They brainstormed and taught them not to tell anyone about their past. In 1994, when their Rebe (spiritual leader) died, they made their followers believe that he was still alive and that their Rebe is the Messiah. In order to keep them interested in their group, and in their beliefs, they send their students to perform good deeds. They party and watch movies of their Rebe. These people are harmless, but they are extremely confused, and they are misleading innocent helpless people. Despite their bizarre beliefs, their followers are the largest group of all other Jewish groups in the world.

Picture one shows a cult while performing rituals. The group sits in a circle close to one another, and members feel a sense of togetherness. Members are opinionless, quiet, and somewhat stoned. They do whatever their leader tells them to do. Painfully, such followers must disconnect from their families and friends and must live by the rules set by their leader. Most people struggle with it. They want to contact their families and friends. But out of fear, they must follow rules.

Picture two shows a pleasant individual who finds some freedom while associating with birds. He or she feels comfort and love from birds. These feelings are mutual. The birds are not necessarily animals, but they could present an absent family connection. Pictures or mementos can fill this void.

Picture three represents a thinker. His or her mind is always preoccupied with bizarre and quite frightening thoughts. This individual is possessed with dreams, his mind wanders, and he has a hard time concentrating.

Picture four shows a need to escape from a current situation, but this individual is so involved with his or her new lifestyle that he is basically drowning in fear and cannot pull himself together and find solutions to return to a normal life. He needs help, but is afraid to ask for it.

THE PERFECT IMAGE

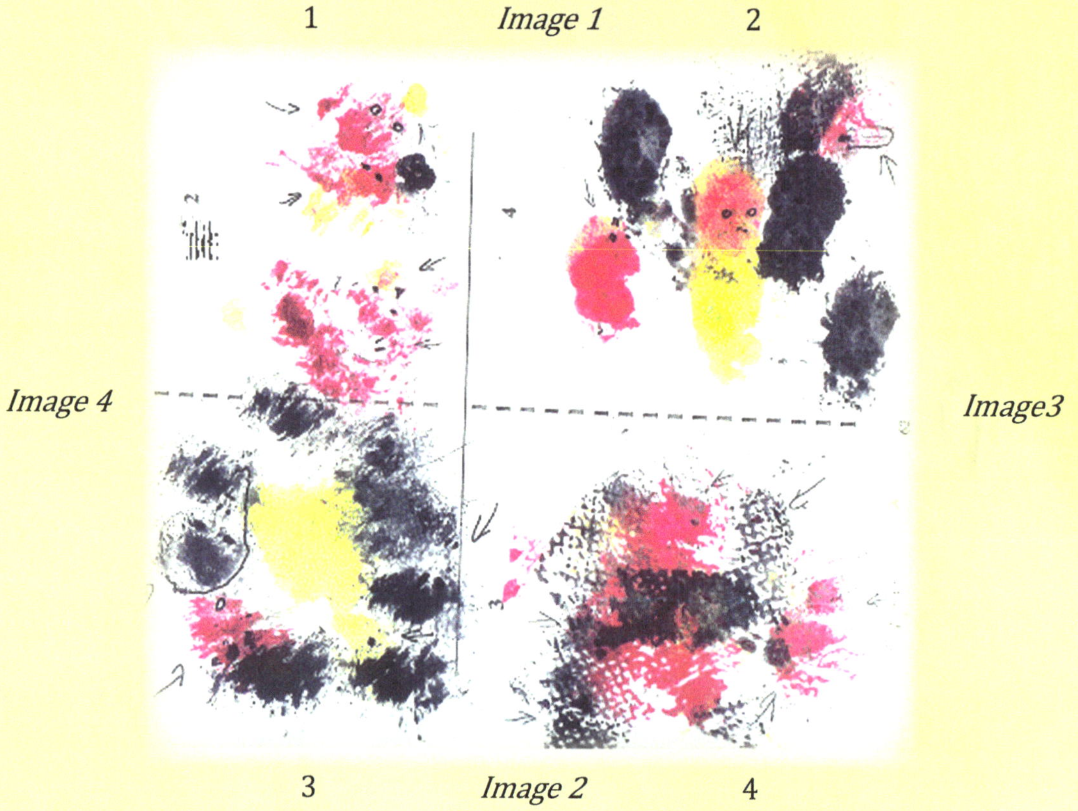

A **perfect image** is when the picture is well defined, and the counselor can get a complete or final reading. If the first draft is clear enough, and the energy is strong enough for the counselor to get the feel of the artist's energy, and it can be read, then there is no need to take an atomic sample. When many issues overwhelm the client, the first draft would most likely not be defined clearly. In such cases, we must take atomic samples until the pictures become clear enough to be read.

For these paintings, the client uses oil paint of choice, cotton balls, cloth, and a sponge. The client may only dip and apply on paper. No water can be used. The perfect image tells the counselor how serious a person is, his goals, imaginations, and how risky he is.

Picture one shows a shy, but risky individual who likes challenges. Most of the time he or she ignores warning signs either because he or she does not understand the danger ahead, or he or she likes to take the risk.

Picture two demonstrates a friendly, outgoing person who takes advantage of his friends to accompany him/her on journeys. Even though his friends go along for the ride, they are skeptical and uncertain of the safety of these trips. Such a person usually likes to visit caves, volcanic sights, post earthquake sights, countries where there are outbreaks of diseases, and other dangerous places.

Picture three shows a harmless person that always ends up in some kind of trouble. Evil people attacking him, falling into mud, or facing natural disasters is very common for him. These incidents are not necessarily related to his adventures. When a person tries to reach out and help, the savior would most likely get trapped in his adventures.

Picture four shows that despite his frequent injuries or troubles, he feels no fear because there are always good Samaritans to bail him out of trouble.

DISCUSSION: The overall picture tells a story of an intelligent, well-educated spectator who wants to study the world. His studies bring great satisfaction to him and to his admirers. Even though his journeys are risky, he is never alone, and he gets enough support from friends and relatives. People are curious, and they are willing to take risks to achieve goals.

LEAD ENERGIZER

PICTURE NINE

The Lead Energizer is designed to diagnose mood disorders, strengths, weaknesses, level of depression, and artistic skills. The lead energizer also acts as a healing tool to remove the spell of evil eyes and mental illness. In this analysis, the client uses a number four pencil if available. If not, a number two pencil will do the job. The client draws in a circular direction and in a restricted area. The client cannot change his mind and erase the drawing. He can scribble as many additional pictures as he wants on another piece of paper. The counselor measures the thickness of the lines, how tight the scribble is, whether there is rhythm of life, or a concern that might affect the client's daily performance. We can also detect whether an individual demonstrates a severe chronic depression, or if there are grounds for his depression and anger.

Image One

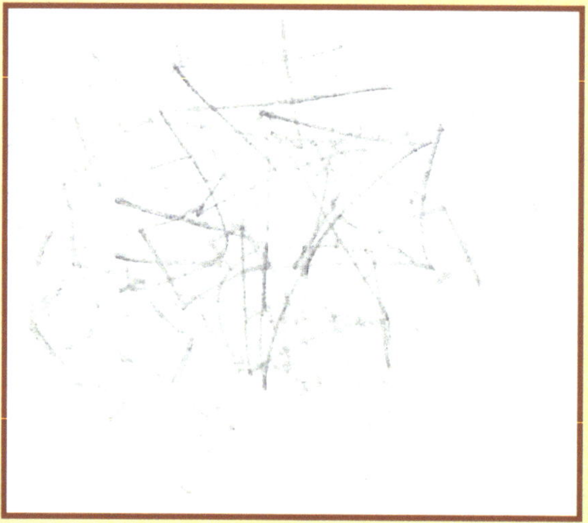

Picture one shows an introvert. The diagram illustrates many little closed squares or boxes with small openings to the center on the left. This indicates that he talks to immediate friends or relatives only when necessary. Nothing extra comes out of his mouth. He is quiet, pleasant, creative, and passive. He is shy and does not share his personal life with others. This person is neither a giver nor a taker. His whole life is about being in his own corner, and seeks no alternatives.

Further, the lines outside are lighter than those in the center. This is a self-centered individual who fears getting involved with the outside world. He is set in his lifestyle. He keeps secrets and never shares any of them with anyone else. Passive and quiet as he is, he cannot be trusted because he does not show any responsibilities or emotions. He feels too comfortable living in isolation. It could be that he was raised in a strict family who did not give him the opportunity to make his own decisions. He had no freedom to speak to outsiders, he could not invite friends, nor does he spend time with friends outside of his home. Education was not important, and everything was catered for him.

Image two

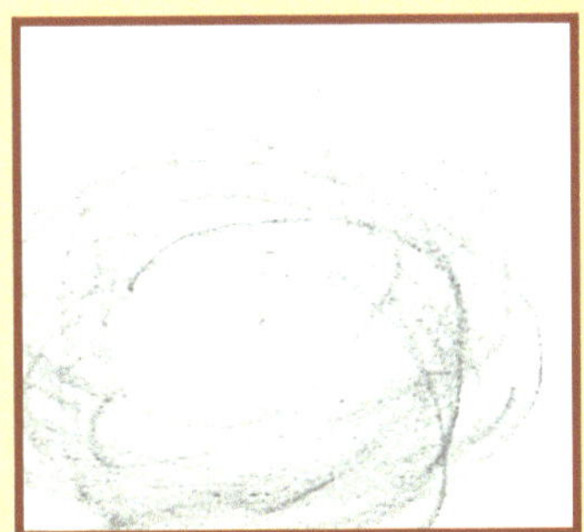

Picture two demonstrates a bowl filled with emotions. There is a dark double line coming up from the center to the right, which indicates that this person is reaching out for help. From the depth of his soul, he feels a void and wants desperately to fill this emptiness. Such characteristics are common in dysfunctional marriages or in a home where there are missing parents. He is seeking freedom, but cannot let go of his past. At this time, however, he tries to escape from his difficulties, but due to his responsibilities, he holds on to a rope he cannot let go of. To the right of the image, there is a tear in the rope. The rip is too far from one end to the next. This indicates that the problem he is in has stretched too far and beyond correction. On the right bottom, we can see a loose rope that is darker than the rest of the drawing. Place your finger on the line and go upward, and see how the line overlaps with a lighter rope. Besides mild overlapping, there are no other knots or loops that seem threatening. The rear of the picture appears like wires or ropes. The front, from the part where the lines overlap, is dark, and it goes all the way to the left. There is a shaded bumpy area, which we call the "ditch of depression." The two lumpy areas show that his depression is not chronic, and he could easily come out of it. On the left bottom, there are loose ropes. One curves to the left and one connects to the right. This person walks through his life as it comes, and deals with each situation separately.

The overall picture suggests the possibility that this client is mourning a loss of a loved one. It could be a spouse, a child, a parent, a friend, a good job, an item, or even the loss of a home.

There are no indications of guilt trips or any emotional complexes that might have triggered his void. This is a loving person who expresses his true inner feelings.

Image three

Picture three shows a diagram of an individual who suffered severe emotional and physical abuse. His whole life is tangled like an animal trapped in a cast iron cage. This person retains lots of anger and does not find room for forgiveness. There is no rhythm of life. To the right, at the edges on top, and on the bottom, there are many edges going in each direction. The lines in the middle are cut short, with reflections of many lighter and darker lines. These suggest a short temper, someone who does not trust anyone, and one who would take revenge to get even. This man is locked in his past and does not know how to move on. This survivor needs a lot of counseling, reassurance, and support as he goes on with life.

Image four

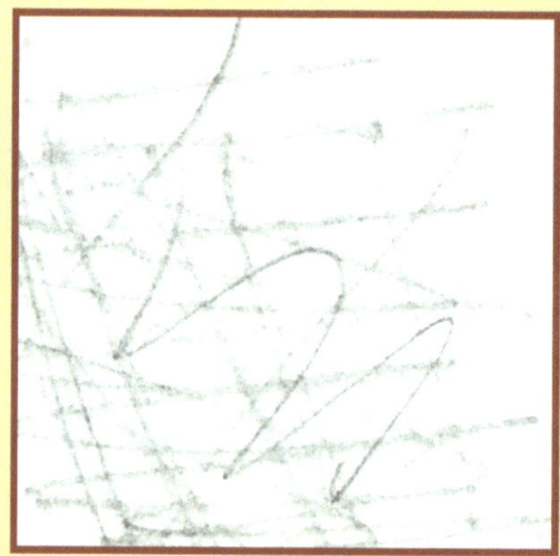

Picture four tells a story of an individual who wishes to express his or her talents but is too shy to proceed with his or her ideas and goals.

Even though the lines seem distorted, most of them are profound and even in color, with a few exceptions in the center. The darker curves show a desire for happiness. If you take a look from a distance, you can see two ladders: one to the left and one geared to the middle. This shows a person with logical goals. On top, in the middle, and on the right, there are loose strings. None of them are knotted, and none of the edges are pointy or sharp. This indicates that this individual is still searching for his desired goals or destinations. The loop on the upper bottom closer to the right indicates that this person holds on to what he already has, before he gets something else. He is a consistent and mature inquirer, anchored, and loves to travel. People find it easy to get along with him, but they don't always trust him because he seems to be forgetful and gets easily sidetracked by thoughts and other stimuli. This individual might still be young and uncertain of how to build his future.

Image five

Image five illustrates a bowl shape. On the left, there are loose wires with one overlapping the other. On the right there is a loose wire with an opening on the bottom. The top does not fit the bowl, and it is sloppy. This is simply a lazy individual who lives a dull life. He has a flat boring personality. He does not smile much and does not get involved in outside affairs. Interestingly, he is open and would travel long distances to meet relatives and friends. He likes to be in the center of affairs, and minds the business of those close to him.

Image six

Picture six illustrates a marvelous creative and learned artist and designer. As we can see, all lines are going to one direction. This demonstrates an organized person that likes to keep everything in order. The colors are reflecting incredible designs and images with messages for the present and the end of times. There is a missing part on the right lower bottom. This corner has no specific messages missing. The missing part on the left bottom is very important for this study. This indicates that he withholds secrets that he is not ready to share with the world. Also, he has some unfinished missions to complete from his past life. The missing parts also suggest that he leaves an open spot to expend his knowledge, and he will eventually bring closure to a story.

This client's portrait tells a story from his past life when he was a writer and an artist. He was also a godly or spiritual figure, and maybe a prophet too. On the top center, there is a hidden date, October 3. The year is not revealed. This date will probably bring great change. I assume that the year of great change will occur in the year 2008 for the following reasons.

1. The end of time has to sum up to (1) in numerology.

2008 2+0+0+8= 10 1+0= (1)

2. The year of great change must include four (0's) and it has to get clustered like cells—which represent a fertilized egg and the beginning of life—the four corners of the world—planets and stars—life, seasons, and environment—heaven—and earth

3. A 0 does not have a beginning and an end.

Except for the number 8 all other numbers from 1- 9 have a beginning and an end. 1, 2, 3, 4, 5, 6, 7, 9

4. We are trapped in a circle with no way to escape just like during childbirth. A baby trapped for nine months in a womb must be born dead or alive.

5. The 8 consist of 2 circles or 2 0's . If you untwist the center of the 8 it will become one big O. The twist in the center symbolizes cells that are progressively forming into one being.

6. At this time we can see many changes in political instability, poor economy, prices and taxes are rising, people lose their homes and businesses, there is going to be many natural disasters such as earthquakes, fires, and other environmental disasters, and wars. We will see more violence and humans and animals will suffer from fear and severe confusion, anger, and depression. We are trying to get away or ignore the situation, but we are trapped, and we must wait patiently for the big tribulation until the end of time.

The artist's present life is on an up and down scale. However, his spiritual strength keeps his morale high. He likes to read the Bible and inexplicable scriptures.

This individual benefits from mystical studies, but does not reveal his extensive knowledge and connection with higher powers. He lives a simple life and knows how to lift up from his troubles with ease. He does not let any obstacles blocking his way.

GEDDI INTERPRETATION

Dr. Goldenthal has performed hundreds of case studies since 1967 with patients, and students of all ages. Based on her findings during art therapy, hypnotherapy, and holistic healing sessions, she devised the Goldenthal Eye Drawing Diagnostic Imaging (GEDDI) test to diagnose and cure persons with Kookshrek Anxiety. She lists some examples of how she interprets images that appear in energy paintings. Some might be universally symbolic while others are individualized. Images change, and they are not always consistent. It depends on how the overall picture appears at the time of the test, and what other images are attached to each picture. For example, when you meet a person for the first time you can tell his height, weight, and maybe get an impression of his personality. Yet when you do business with this gentleman, you might find that he is not honest. The GEDDI is not built on one angle of a person's personality. It involves an overall picture of his mental status, physical health, spirit and soul. If part of an apple rots, you might either throw out the apple, or cut the rotten piece away, and eat the rest. Humans are not the same. If a person's leg rots, it has to be amputated; and the person becomes disabled for life. A missing leg could destroy a victim's spirit, and could have a significant impact on those around him. Persons with disabilities often become dependent on others for physical, emotional, and spiritual support. Therefore, a person must be analyzed as a whole being. In order for the counselor to give the right diagnoses and treat the client properly, he or she must perform a complete analysis. People are sensitive, and we must never judge or label anyone falsely.

A mezuzah (Heb.: doorpost), symbolizes a constant reminder of God's presence and mitzvoth. It also symbolizes the night of Passover in Egypt when God told the Jewish people to smear blood on the doorpost so that the Angel of Death would pass their homes when He killed the first-born Egyptians. In the GEDDI, the mezuzah symbolizes a division between the free world, to a secured sanctuary. A person that comes from the outside and sees a mezuzah on a doorpost feels an instant change. He comes from the open to a secluded protective world.

A cave in the GEDDI symbolizes the beginning of life, the end of a road, a final destination, a holy sanctuary; and a place of comfort.

The cross in Christianity symbolizes the crucifixion of Jesus and a religious symbolic ornament. In the GEDDI, the cross symbolizes tension, uncertainty, and fear to express oneself, a choking sensation that could mean financial struggle.

The Fish in the GEDDI symbolizes a pleasant, kind, modest, helpful, God fearing, and righteous. Fish with teeth symbolizes a modest, but aggressive, angry, and unforgiving individual. He likes to eat junk food and does not care about his health. Yet he is sharp, has good common sense, is a good businessman, and is financially settled. He manages well. He does not allow anyone to trick him, cheat, or mislead him.

The menorah is a seven-branched candelabrum and is a symbol of the Jewish nation. (Isaiah 42:6).

A Yarmulka or skullcap comes from the Aramaic word "yerai malka" (fear of or respect for the King). The custom in Western cultures is the opposite; it symbolizes respect to remove one's hat.

The Magen David or the Star of David is relatively new and symbolically associated with Judaism today. It also represents the shape of King David's shield. Today, the Magen David is a universally recognized symbol of Jewry. It appears on the flag of the state of Israel, and the Israeli equivalent of the Red Cross is known as the Red Magen David.

The Flag in the GEDDI represents one that feels comfortable in his present situation. He does not like changes, does not like to share with outsiders, prefers to keep to himself, is overprotective, selective of friends, and does not trust strangers.

The flag universally symbolizes different meanings. From earliest recorded history, flags were used for ceremonies, war, territories, and symbols of nations. For example:

A white flag signified a request for surrender.

A red flag symbolizes warnings.

A black flag symbolizes stormy oceans.

A red cross signified a place of neutral immunity.

Army legions would fly a standard flag as a symbol of nation independence.

In the Bible, flags are mentioned many times after the exodus of the Israelites from Egypt. Every tribe had a flag with its own color. The Bible also relates. "And the Children of Israel shall encamp, each man in his own camp, and every man by his own flag, throughout their hosts . . . and thus they encamped according to their flags and thus they journeyed each man with his family according to his fathers house" *(Numbers 1:52; 2:34).*

G-d commanded Moses to make flags for the tribes of Israel. As soon as they were settled, they blew their trumpets and Judah and his flag moved first, followed by the prince and his tribe" *(Numbers, Midrash Tanhuma 2).*

According to this Midrash, the flags of the tribes were of the same color as the stones of Aaron the High Priests breastplate. There were twelve precious stones on the breastplate arranged in four rows, with three stones in each row. Altogether there were twelve different stones in varied colors, and according to the color everyone would know the color of the flag of his tribe. In the consciousness of the people of Israel, the Shield of David symbolizes hope in the future, and a star that will brighten the heavens. According to the Jewish thinker, Franz Rosenzweig (1886-1929), the six-pointed Shield of David represents the creation, the revelation of G-d as the final redemption.

Standing horse: in the GEDDI it symbolizes kindness, politeness, affectionate, caring, carries out tasks in a timely manner, a good listener, one who likes to learn and is giving.

Running horse: zestful, has a rhythm or tempo to life, cheerful, outgoing, likes to party, has a short attention span, likes to be on top of things, is always in need to keep busy, and somewhat aggressive and even scheming. Likes to reach out to the needy, needs to be appreciated and recognized, has strong leadership skills, but does not like to take commands from others.

Standing up horse on two feet: represents an affectionate, cheer leader, sporty, playful person who likes to laugh, comical, nudges, gets what he wants, gets easily insulted, forgives easily, likes a specific lifestyle, well organized, very creative, likes people to listen to him/her, but hates to take commands or advice from others.

Reversed image: two human faces represent a hypocrite, someone deceitful, and untrusting. He likes to promise but never delivers his promise, interferes, minds someone else's business, is jealous, unhappy with his looks, and thinks someone else has more than him/her.

Dual image, one side human and one side animal: Immature, restless, undecided, needs guidance and reminders, withdrawn, unexpressive, responds slowly, always on the run, requires constant reassurance, needs to be loved, likes to give, preserves his self-worth, cheats on spouse, friends and co-workers, lacks feelings for others, has low self-esteem, hostile, cries easily, is disruptive, tends to smoke and drink. He hits, but always apologizes.

Turtle-in shell- shy, learning disabled, withdrawn, scared, quiet, feels comfortable in isolation, giving, charitable, modest, good housekeeper and provider, not searching for attention, likes to learn new skills. Can also be sneaky and unpredictable.

Turtle, out of shell: modest, conservative, likes to teach and learn, good listener, open-minded, looks up to peers, respectful, easy going, tends to be controlled and manipulated by others, has difficulty expressing himself, does not enjoy intimate relationships, sociable, not informative, slow learner, afraid of commitments, keeps to himself, can be rich, but prefers to live simple.

Birds - freedom, unsettled, little concern for others, spontaneous, gives up easily, relies on others, full of excuses, talks too much, travels, likes to visit historic and modern-sights, hates to read, learns from life experience, hates to be structured.

Images of cartoons-If the cartoon appears in the circle of the picture, he is outgoing, likes to show off his artistic talents, articulated, and expressive. If the sample of his personality is out of range, he is somewhat dull, not aware of his talent, a con-artist, introvert, feels comfortable with familiar people only, insecure, does not trust others, truthful with himself, unaffectionate, happy but not expressive, needs directions, acts like an automat rather than human.

Strikes - (x) indicates rage, hopelessness, unhappiness, emotionally unbalanced, instability, tends to blame others for their evil behavior.

Fish-spontaneous, loveable, affectionate, modest, pleasant, enjoys life and nature. Gets along easily, has a good rhythm of life, educated, appreciative, but defenseless when out of his ordinary life. Likes his own environment and surroundings.

Figures-in a circle- strong desire to belong, needs instructions and reassurance, follower, rebellious, easily manipulated, susceptible to brainstorming, usually not aware when hurting others by his bizarre behavior, not aware of community norms, strong belief in rituals, feels unloved at home and reaches out to others for love.

Figures-out of a circle-Likes to be known, flexible, smokes and drinks for showoff, likes to interact with small groups, hates lectures, usually not learned and illiterate. He is a hard workingman, pretends to be a millionaire, likes to impress strangers, and hates to help his family. A person like this is often cheating on his spouse and separates or divorces.

Water-flow of income, richness, earns sufficient money, expressive, sophisticated, tends to share feelings, open to meet new friends, periods of mood swings, rage, and blows out of proportion. Tends to calm down, forgive, and go on with life.

Drowning-financial ruin, wobbly, reserved, dysfunctional, gives up easily, antisocial, does not trust other people, no self-confidence, depressed, recognizes situations,

deals with them alone, and avoids reaching out for help or guidance.

Rain-New hope, new growth, charitable, tends to help and guide friends.

Puddles-easily angered, health issues, fails unless willing to seek professional help, likes sports, does not like guidance; possibly depressed.

Fog - fearful, has difficulties in decision making, unset mind, thinks a lot prior to proceeding with a plan or project, takes extra precautions, must know a person well before committing a friendship, loner, depressed, isolated, does not know how to reach out to people, prefers not to be troubled.

Snake - Intelligent, gets what he wants, achiever, goal oriented, sexual dominator, minds someone else's business, controller, trustless, con artist.

Metal - stubborn, aggressive, and needs to control. Committed to decisions, keeps his job, stable, good businessman, strong family ties, good provider, well educated, has a hard time forgiving when lied to or cheated on, anticipates positive outcomes even during difficult times, has good control over children, his word must be respected, attractive to weaker women, makes a good inspector, judges, likes to teach and be a community leader.

Star - Good leadership and management skills, controlling, always on top of things, kind, positive attitude, good hearted, likes to share, outspoken, smiles a lot, groomed well, likes peace.

Boat - loaner, minds own business, likes music, gets easily depressed, fantasizes, creative, hates routines, loves nature, spiritually connected to G-d, but his faith fluctuates with his mood swings.

Airplane - enjoys challenges, tends to escape from responsibilities, needs freedom, loves to play volleyball, soccer, tennis, and basketball. Worries a lot, restless, cannot stay in one place for too long, spontaneous, sociable, and good businessperson.

Alligator - good guard, strong positive attitude, provider, likes to eat junk food, somewhat lazy, positive self-image, deceitful, good listener but slow learner, con-artist, jealous of someone else's possessions, usually rich without effort, doesn't require much education to survive, likes gambling or risking, has difficulty making decisions, needs guidance, lacks common sense, tends to make frequent mistakes, has short stays in jail, self centered, and fails to see obstacles around him.

Duck - very warm and loving, somewhat a yenta, easygoing, proud of himself, positive outlook on life, overprotective, nurturing, religious, likes to share, good provider, observant, slow to trust strangers.

Bushes - personality disorder, tricky, natural, likes to explode, growth, observant, likes enhancement, loyal to job and family responsibilities, frequent mood swings with frequent outbursts.

Square shaped house - content, safeguarded, builds many goals but does not fulfill them, middle class, likes to argue, must be heard, somewhat controlling, likes to impress others rather than own family, hostile, open to learn new skills, likes a neat home but expects someone else to do it, unorganized at home and financially, forgives easily.

Square raised roof home with an attic - dangerous, rich, possibly haunted, tends to have tragedies such as death, physical and emotional ailments, lies, refuses to share secrets, ego conflict, domineering, often troubled with the law, conflict with family, like hunting, paintings, music, desires to be known, yet shies away from society.

Fire - cozy, warm, high tempered, argumentative, hurries to spread news, tends to shoplift, projects his faults on others, ego centered, authoritarian, good learner, usually academically inclined, and a good speaker.

Window - likes to air out feelings to neighbors and friends, minds someone else's business, very clean, well organized, likes to help, well known in community, straight forward, likes to connect to the universe, likes to volunteer, speaks without considering others feelings, likes to attend meetings and travel.

www.ingramcontent.com/pod-product-compliance
Ingram Content Group UK Ltd.
Pitfield, Milton Keynes, MK11 3LW, UK
UKHW060119300726
14090UKWH00002B/269
* 9 7 8 1 4 3 6 3 3 2 1 6 3 *